CW01213263

Rapid Weight Loss Hypnosis Guidebook

A Transforming Guide On Weight Loss With Self-Hypnosis And Meditation To Stop Emotional Eating And Learn Healthy Mini Habits To Increase Your Self-Esteem

Madeline J.Cox

Rapid Weight Loss Hypnosis Crash Course

Rapid Weight Loss Hypnosis Crash Course

©Copyright 2021 All rights reserved.

This document is geared towards providing exact and reliable information in regards to the topic and issue covered. The publication is sold with the idea that the publisher is not required to render accounting, officially permitted or otherwise qualified services. If advice is necessary, legal or professional, a practiced individual in the profession should be ordered.

From a Declaration of Principles which was accepted and approved equally by a Committee of the American Bar Association and a Committee of Publishers and Associations.

In no way is it legal to reproduce, duplicate, or transmit any part of this document in either electronic means or in printed format. Recording of this publication is strictly prohibited, and any storage of this document is not allowed unless with written permission from the publisher. All rights reserved.

The information provided herein is stated to be truthful and consistent, in that any liability, in terms of inattention or otherwise, by any usage or abuse of any policies, processes, or directions contained within is the solitary and utter responsibility of the recipient reader. Under no circumstances will any legal responsibility or blame be held against the publisher for any reparation, damages, or monetary loss due to the information herein, either directly or indirectly.

Respective authors own all copyrights not held by the publisher.

The information herein is offered for informational purposes solely and is universal as so. The presentation of the information is without a contract or any type of guarantee assurance.

The trademarks used are without any consent, and the publication of the trademark is without permission or backing by the trademark owner. All trademarks and brands within this book are for clarifying purposes only and are owned by the owners themselves, not affiliated with this document.

Rapid Weight Loss Hypnosis Crash Course

Table of Contents

INTRODUCTION 8

CHAPTER 1: HOW HYPNOSIS WORK: OVERPOWERED AND OUT OF CONTROL 12

    Prepared to Eat Wrong 13

    The Brain Cares How You Feel 15

CHAPTER 2: BASICS OF MEDITATION 20

    How to Prepare 21

        The Right Ambience 22

        Right Posture 22

        Breathing Exercises and Tips 22

        Now That You Are Ready, What Are You Going to Do? 24

CHAPTER 3: BODY IMAGE RELAXATION 26

    How to Perform Body Image Meditation 27

CHAPTER 4: POWER OF SELF-CONFIDENCE 30

    Self-Confidence 30

        Meditation for Self-Confidence 31

    Self-Love 32

        Meditation for Self-Love 32

CHAPTER 5: PLEASURE PRINCIPLE 36

    Wired for Flavor 37

        The Physics of Flavor 39

CHAPTER 6: EATING OUT ON EFFECTIVE WEIGHT LOSS PROGRAM 44

Specific Rules for Eating Out 45
The Rules of Working Out 49

CHAPTER 7: FOODS TO EAT FOR DEEPER MEDITATION 52

Affirmations to Heal Your Food Relationship 55

CHAPTER 8: THE FOUR GOLDEN RULES 58

Golden Rule One - When You Are Hungry, Eat! 58
Recognizing Real Hunger 59
The Hunger Scale 61
Golden Rule Two - Eat What You Want, Not What You Think You Should 62
Golden Rule Three - Whenever You Eat, Do It Consciously 63
Concentrate on Your Food 64

CHAPTER 9: THE PSYCHOLOGY ABOUT WEIGHT LOSS 66

Weight Loss Is Hard 66
Don't Let Fears Hold You Back 68

CHAPTER 10: THE SECRET TO GETTING RID OF WEIGHT PROBLEMS 74

Weight Loss Affirmations: Are They Enough and How to Practice Them 78
Creative Visualization 80

CHAPTER 11: CONDITION FOR HYPNOSIS TO WORK OUT 82

Motivation 83
Optimism 83
Defending 83
Concentration 84

- *Acceptability* *84*
- *Imagination* *85*

CHAPTER 12: YOUR THINNER AND HAPPIER LIFE **88**
- BENEFITS OF EATING HEALTHY AND DETOXIFYING 88
  - *Maintain a Healthy Body* *89*
  - *Maintain the Bodyweight* *90*

CONCLUSION **96**

Rapid Weight Loss Hypnosis Crash Course

Introduction

Many audio packs provided by professional hypnotherapists have the very same session on CD or MP3 and are much less costly as the hypnotherapist only has to record the session once with certain clients.

And if you're talking about gastric band surgery, the natural form of hypnotherapy may well be worth your consideration.

Hypnotic Gastric Banding Therapy

The therapist opens the subconscious mind to feedback and attempts not to change an old pattern, but to create a new one.

The hypnotherapist will indicate to your subconscious mind that you simply have a stomach-fitted surgical band and that your stomach is just the size of a golf ball. The hypnotherapist should speak to you about the process.

Your experience will begin with the therapist bringing you through a very calm state of mind, and you are led through all the sounds of the hospital that one would expect to hear, such as the voices and noises wheeling down the hospital's corridors on the way to the operating theatre.

You must move through in-hospital doctors and nurses, bangs and clangs of sterile stainless-steel bowls and instruments, and a bustling metropolitan hospital's general everyday noise.

The gurney (operating trolley) then stops when you enter the operating room, and the nurse asks if you are ready for surgery. You respond "Yes," so the anesthetist moves forward to administer anesthetic.

You can hear people talking about the operation of the gastric band, you can hear alarms beeping, and you feel surgically operated on. The hypnotic banding weight loss treatment takes you through the whole surgical cycle.

Gastric band surgery, as you probably already know, is a common weight loss choice. Many very overweight and obese individuals underwent surgery and lost hundreds of pounds and kilos successfully. Hypnosis-assisted weight loss is another choice for Gastric Lap Band Surgery.

Patients who have undergone the hypnotic version feel that they've actually had the surgery, as I mentioned many of them even raise their shirts to see if they've had an incision after the surgery they think they've just had, the hypnotherapist's thought deep inside their subconscious is so strong that people find it hard to believe they haven't.

Hypnotic gastric banding or weight loss with hypnosis support is pain-free and also a healthy way to have gastric band surgery. There is an alternative to spending significant sums of money on surgery, and the sometimes-prolonged recovery period is not required. You have all the surgery advantages, but without the complications.

As many TV shows feature them, Hypnotic Gastric Banding is increasingly common. Hypnosis weight loss is a fantastic option and many clients will testify to having lost hundreds of pounds from this type of therapy.

Enjoy opening your mind and discovering life's various possibilities. Hypnotherapy is now commonly recognized and is growing as the impressive outcomes become more well-known and more physicians, many in the medical community and natural therapists see and support the therapies available using hypnotherapy.

CHAPTER 1:
How Hypnosis Work: Overpowered and Out of Control

I'm continually contemplating nourishment and attempting to shed pounds," Mary said during her first session. "It works for some time, however then I become weary of it. Something consistently occurs and disrupts the general flow.

At that point, I restore all the weight, in addition to another 10 pounds for the most part. I commit dumb errors, and I'm sluggish. I simply don't want to work out. It appears as though I harm myself. I don't have the foggiest idea of what else to do."

This sort of reasoning is normal for individuals who battle to shed pounds and keep it off - the negative self-talk, believing they're self-attacking, or there is a major issue with them — and who can accuse them? By and large, they've pursued each arrangement, done all that they "thought" they should do — despite everything it didn't work.

What they don't understand is that there are parts of science and how the brain really functions at play here, and by getting familiar with how the psyche really functions, the things that used to be keeping them down would now be able to assist them with being effective.

Prepared to Eat Wrong

We are prepared since early on to treat nourishment with a specific goal in mind. When we're little youngsters, we're frequently advised to "finish all the nourishment on your plate," or "would prefer you not to grow up huge and solid?" Huge numbers of these benevolent proclamations made by grown-ups are really neutralizing our science — supposing that you see how kids eat, you'll see they'd frequently prefer to play over eat.

They're increasingly keen on investigating their general surroundings, playing with their toys and different children than eating, on the off chance that they're not really ravenous.

At that point as we get more established, we're instructed that "breakfast is the most significant meal of the day," and much of the time we're not permitted to venture out from home without eating a "decent breakfast." Lunch is at a particular time each day, so we need to eat at that point or not in any way. This frequently proceeds into adulthood where at work, we make some specific memories edge to have lunch, are as yet having breakfast toward the beginning of the day, regardless of whether we're really eager or not.

We're encouraged that nourishment is there to assist us with feeling better, "eat something and you'll feel good." We go out for dessert when we win the softball match-up, and go out for pizza when our rabbit kicks the bucket. Without our rabbit kicks the bucket. Without acknowledging it, our social reactions to nourishment are instructing us to sincerely eat.

The issue with these components that are a piece of our general public is that it's not quite we as people are structured. We have something many refer to as a craving. Our craving is the body's regular method to disclose to us when it's a great opportunity to eat, or when it's an ideal opportunity to quit eating.

What's more, we're prepared out of utilizing our craving at a youthful age by being compelled to eat at explicit occasions, or eat explicit measures of nourishment when we're not ravenous. Contrast that with other basic substantial capacities — like realizing when to go to the restroom, for instance.

Ask yourself — how would you realize when it's a great opportunity to go to the restroom? Do you plan it? Do you plan it, and consider it throughout the day? Most likely not .

Probably the most ideal ways we can gain power back with regards to eating, is to give the activity of realizing when it's a great opportunity to eat and what amount back to the body, and away from the reasoning procedure. This is tied in with returning to the genuine power that we're brought into the world with - our bodies' own intelligence incorporated with a significant part of our body called our craving, and start eating when our body reveals to us it's a great opportunity to eat and stop when we're fulfilled or full.

It's called Mindful Eating, and it's conceivable to begin utilizing our hunger again to assist us with accomplishing the weight reduction we want. Regardless of whether you don't think you have a hunger - you may astonish yourself. Numerous customers have revealed some fear when it came to utilizing their craving to help manage their nourishment consumption, since they state they don't really have a hunger and aren't sure in the event that they realize when they're fulfilled or full. What's more, it might be valid — meds and ailment are two things that can affect our feeling of craving. Be that as it may, I generally ask them to simply attempt it — hold up until they're eager to eat and see what occurs.

What's more, for each situation, customers are astonished to learn they do in reality have a craving, and it can help direct their nourishment utilization. Careful Eating implies you utilize your hunger to eat when you're eager and stop when you're full, eating well nourishment in sound parcels.

The Brain Cares How You Feel

The other component keeping individuals caught in weight gain is the mind's characteristic propensity to get some distance from torment and toward delight.

There's a lot of logical foundation on how this functions, yet to streamline it, there are two contending portions of our mind that are continually attempting to help keep us sheltered and upbeat.

One is the limbic framework. It's a more established, progressively crude piece of our mind. The essential focal point of this piece of the mind is to protect us. It reacts to feelings and inspiration, is answerable for long haul memory, and it doesn't prefer to feel agitated or uncertain in light of the fact that those sentiments are dangerous.

Be that as it may, we as a whole realize we live in a universe of vulnerability, so the limbic framework is regularly miserable. When something transpires that we don't care for - for instance, we're exhausted, or tragic, or upset, this piece of the mind feels awkward, and the characteristic propensity is for this piece of the cerebrum to get us to improve. This is the place numerous individuals stumble into difficulty, since when feeling exhausted or focused on, nourishment will frequently fill in as a generally excellent distractor to offer some relief. The cerebrum is glad - quickly, on the grounds that nourishment gives prompt delight.

The issue is that it's likewise fleeting, so with the goal for you to really feel much improved, you'll need to continue eating. This is the manner by which a whole sack of treats vanishes and how we eat more than we need, which thusly can make us put on weight.

The other piece of the mind at work here is the prefrontal cortex. This piece of the mind is the fresher, official capacity part of the cerebrum liable for long haul arranging. This is the piece of the mind that realizes it's bad to eat a whole pack of treats and wouldn't like to eat the whole sack either.

So the issue is that with these two contending portions of our mind at play, we regularly feel clashed — with part of us needing to eat the treats to feel better now, and part of us realizing we'll think twice about it later.

Furthermore, the genuine test comes in light of the fact that the nourishment really improves.

All in all, the limbic piece of the mind is really relieved by the nourishment. So truly the nourishment attempts to assist us with feeling much improved — however, it's just an impermanent arrangement — we feel better just while we're really eating. Over the long haul eating for enthusiastic reasons transforms into an unfortunate propensity and causes weight gain.

The explanation this is imperative to comprehend is that there is a superior way. The limbic framework doesn't really require nourishment — it simply needs to feel much improved, and there are numerous different things that will make this piece of the mind feel good.

The issue is that nourishment works so well in the transient that numerous individuals depend upon it only — so when the opportunity arrives, and we are not feeling better, we just have one reaction. What's more, that is to eat something. At that point, we feel wild.

The initial phase in any change procedure is mindfulness.

What's more, for a considerable lot of my customers just understanding this is the means by which the mind works — the explanation you go after nourishment when you feel exhausted, focused, miserable, and blameworthy is that there's a piece of your cerebrum that simply needs you to feel good — simply realizing that the procedure is mostly the cerebrum normal reaction, that can assist us with settling on a superior decision since we understand there's nothing amiss with us.

For Mary, she understood that in the event that she just took a full breath, and ventured outside, she could regularly evade the automatic reaction to passionate triggers in her day-by-day life. This gave her a quick feeling of control, regardless of whether it was just a piece of the time from the outset.

In any case, gradually, after some time, the mind starts to overhaul itself. Presently, rather than simply having a solitary alternative to feel much improved nourishment, there are various choices: a walk, tea, call a companion, tune in to music. Furthermore, with those numerous decisions comes a significant part of making change: the delay. A minute to stop, reflect, and really pick the manner in which you react to a circumstance so you can get the outcomes you need.

CHAPTER 2:
Basics of Meditation

Meditation is the art of quieting the mind. It is the art of awakening our consciousness. Meditation helps us shift from a consciousness bound by a small ego to a deeper sense of self. We will achieve peace of mind, relaxation, and a positive attitude about ourselves and the world if we meditate properly. When we have a healthy mind and an increased self-esteem, the rest of our being will benefit too. We will find better health when we reduce our tension, and we can be comfortable no matter what life throws at us.

Meditation practice is mostly used as a part of meditation and other metaphysical disciplines. Some of the benefits are that you do not need any special equipment or location to do meditation .

The basic concepts of meditation are similar, there are several ways in which it can be performed. The most important, and sometimes the hardest part is to relax your mind and avoid following any distracting wandering thoughts.

It is the negative thoughts which are polluting the mind. You will find harmony and relaxation in a hectic day, by learning to keep them out. Training to keep your mind quiet helps you to concentrate on deeper, more positive thoughts that motivate you to enjoy life more.

When you trudge down life's fatiguing alleys, life always resembles a rat race. Workplace tension, frustration at home and intense soul fatigue add up to build a peculiar state. Sometimes the busy workers thought they had handled their lives better if the day had 36 or more hours in it. Yet, there are several risks that arise from persistent stress and anxiety. Indeed, almost all modern illnesses are somehow connected to the stressful lifestyle. Meditating is the best way to counter the fatigue and tiredness.

Now meditation will only produce great replenishing results if you do it in the right way. Too many people know meditation's common benefits, but very few know how to meditate. If this is the first time that you intend to engage in any meditation exercises, it is recommended that you meet with a qualified trainer or someone who is experienced in such techniques. Here are a few basics of meditation for beginners to support.

How to Prepare

You need to make some arrangements before meditating. At first, try to secure in the early morning at some time. The explanation for this is that a person is usually in his best mood and health in the morning. You should perform this exercise with an empty stomach. And if you prefer meditation evening, make sure you did not take any food at least three hours before the session. Taking a cool shower before meditating is always healthy. This will help you to concentrate better .

The Right Ambience

You need a great ambience for proper meditation, which is serene and calm. Choose a place to get yourself some solitude. Mild, calming fragrance would be of great help in this. Space light should be dim, and the session should not be disturbed by noise.

Right Posture

Posture is also an essential factor influencing the action. With a sitting position or lying position, you can do it all. Yet the beginners also fall asleep while they are lying on the floor or mattress doing this. Hence beginning with a sitting posture is advisable.

The typical method of meditating is to sit cross beamed on a mat or a flat mattress in a posture called Lotus. But if you have knee pain or other discomforts, consider sitting on a chair that holds the back and neck straight.

Breathing Exercises and Tips

Few special breathing techniques that are mandatory at the time of the sessions. Deep breathing is one of the most common meditation techniques, where both the process of inhalation and exhalation is long and slow. You should try to focus on thinking about one specific thing. Besides these, there are other strategies that you can get from any book or other tools on "How to Meditate."

Meditation is the best way to calm your mind and rejuvenate the damage to your soul as well. Practice it daily and track the results over a short period.

Below are a few tips to help you learn to practice the art of meditation.

Bring some comfortable clothing on first. Close-fitting trousers and tight clothes are likely to be something of a nuisance. Find something to wear that lets you relax without having to worry about being pinched or pulled.

You can then play some good and calming instrumental music. If you listen to music with lyrics when you are meditating, you are likely to start singing along in your ear, which will not help you concentrate.

To help them concentrate, some people think it helps to have a candle or other item to look at. Many tend to close their eyes to help avoid anything that might disrupt their mental comfort.

Sit in a snug spot. Putting a pillow under your bottom could help you sit up straight and balanced. When you think you can stay awake during your meditation period, you can always lie in bed or on the couch. What is crucial is that the place helps you to relax as you concentrate.

The position or location may also be helpful. Select a place that is free from disturbance inside your home.

A place where temperature and appearance are both relaxed and friendly. There are those who decorate a specific part of a room only for meditation purposes.

Switch your mobile phone off the Screen and the ringer. You may want to set the timer on your phone, so you will know when it is time to stop without having to check every minute to see how long it has been. If this is a new activity for you, simply schedule it for 5 minutes and start developing your meditation skills. As you develop your ability to concentrate and quiet your mind, you can extend your meditation practice.

Now That You Are Ready, What Are You Going to Do?

There are two rising meditation methods. One focuses on the air, during mindfulness instruction that is also a technique taught. You just focus on the air as you inhale through your nose and softly exhale through your mouth. Reflect on the wind feeling when it gets into the body. See it as it moves through your lungs, giving life to your mind and then see it as it leaves your body .

Any time an outside thought comes into your mind, accept it but do not act on it, just return your attention to your breath for the time that you set it.

The other common approach is to imagine a healing beam of light that hits your eyes, bringing to your mind and body a wave of relaxation and peace. Let it search gently across your body, starting at your head and slowly going all the way to the tips of your toes. When you feel any stress or discomfort, just imagine the soothing beam that dissolves discomfort and stress in your body.

There is really no downside to meditation practice. No physical exertion or special equipment is required. If you have any mobility problems, just sit in a chair providing you with the support you need to feel secure and relaxed.

Meditation has been shown to relieve tension and to be helpful in many ways, such as changing a person's outlook on life. It is easy to do, and yet difficult because at the same time, you are learning to relax and control your thoughts. Take 5 minutes a day and do a week or two of meditation practice. You can do it for free, and the benefits you get will significantly improve your life!

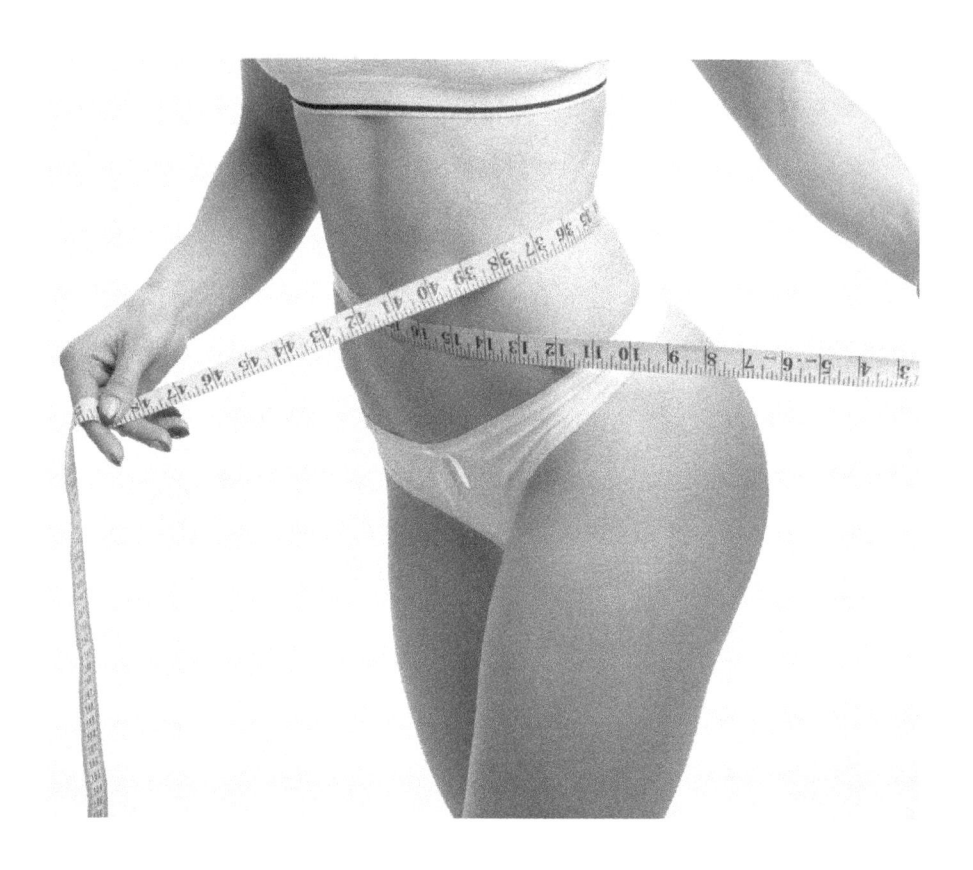

CHAPTER 3:
Body Image Relaxation

Body image meditation helps reduce stress by making you aware of how your body feels instead of paying attention to stressful thoughts.

When you feel stressed out, your body also feels those effects, and it starts to show signs of stress through pain in your back, stomach or tensed shoulders.

You may even experience neck ache, particularly if you have been concentrating on things that were difficult and that strained you in some way.

You may just have aching bones because you are cold or because you feel worn out in general, but a body image can help you to feel much better.

By practicing body image meditation, you distract your mind from the stressful thoughts by paying attention to those parts of the body that feel stressed.

As a result, you become mindful of your body and forgetful of the thoughts that bring you stress. Thus, you feel relaxed and your stress levels greatly reduce.

Here is a step-by-step guide on how you can perform this meditation technique.

How to Perform Body Image Meditation

The first step is to find a quiet place to perform this meditation technique, which is similar to the other techniques that I have mentioned earlier. Once you are in a quiet place with no distractions, then follow the steps mentioned below:

- Lie on your back on the floor in a position that makes you feel comfortable. Make sure that your posture doesn't make you uncomfortable. If lying on the floor hurts, then you can lie on a mattress or bed instead; there is no hard and fast rule that you have to lie on the floor.

The aim here for you is to feel comfortable. You can slide a pillow under your back if you feel uneasy or you can lie on your side: right or left—whichever makes you feel relaxed. The preferred position is on your back using only one pillow to support your head so that your airways are clear.

- As soon as you settle, take a deep breath to calm your racing mind. Sometimes, it may take you longer than just one deep breath, depending on how your day went. If that's the case, keep breathing deeply until you feel a sense of calmness in your mind. A great way to calm your racing mind is to focus on the breath as you take it. In fact, if it helps you, use the counting that you used before—8 for the inhale through the nostrils and 10 for the exhale. You can even see if you are breathing deeply enough by placing a hand on your upper abdomen and feeling it going up when you breathe in and down when you exhale.

- Once your mind is calm, bring your attention to your body. Feel every sensation in it. Start with the tingling feeling in your toes and feet. Once you feel it, slowly shift your attention from your feet to other parts of your body.

Feel the tension in each part as you move up from your toes to your head.

Feel the tension in the muscles of your legs and the sensations in your belly or the tension in your shoulders and back, depending on where you feel the most stress and pain. Feel the strain in your head, and your eyelids hurt as you open and close them .

Note: In the process of examining every sensation in your body, your mind will try to distract you by bringing in different thoughts. If that happens, bring your focus back to your body and start again from the toes and slowly move up to the head and try again to feel the tension on each part. If it helps you at all, I find that being conscious of that area of the body, followed by tensing the area and then purposely relaxing it helps a lot. As you relax that part of the body, feel the weight as the body relaxes.

- Do this exercise for 15–20 minutes at the start and then slowly increase the time as you get good at it. Remember that your mind is your

#1 enemy, as it keeps distracting you from bringing in countless thoughts that only end up causing stress and anxiety. However, you have to fight it (which is a continuous struggle); with time and patience, everything can be achieved.

- Body image meditation is hard as compared to the other techniques that I have mentioned before but, if done properly, it is a great technique, as it can greatly help you to relieve stress and anxiety almost instantly. It also helps to lower your blood pressure and bring your heartbeat down, so do remember to get up slowly from the exercise and relax for a moment before going into your everyday activities again.

So far, you have learnt three of the most effective meditation techniques to reduce stress and anxiety. To get better results, it is important to enhance their effectiveness.

CHAPTER 4:
Power of Self-Confidence

Self-love is probably the best thing you can accomplish for yourself. Being infatuated with yourself furnishes you with fearlessness, self-esteem and it will, by and large, help you feel progressively positive.

You may likewise find that it is simpler for you to experience passionate feelings for once you have found out how to cherish yourself first. On the off chance that you can find out how to adore yourself, you will be a lot more joyful and will find out how to best deal with yourself, paying little respect to the circumstance you are in.

Self-Confidence

Self-confidence is just the demonstration of putting a standard in oneself. Believing in yourself is one of the most significant ethics to develop so as to make your mind powerful.

Fearlessness likewise realizes more bliss. Regularly, when you are sure about your capacities, you are more joyful because of your triumphs. When you are resting easy thinking about your abilities, the more stimulated and inspired you are to make a move and accomplish your objectives.

Meditation for Self-Confidence

Sit easily and close your eyes. Count from 1 to 5, concentrating on your breath as you breathe as it were of quiet and unwinding through your nose and breathe out totally through your mouth. Experience yourself as progressively loose and quiet, prepared to extend your experience of certainty and prosperity right now. Proceeding to concentrate on your breath, breathing one might say of quiet, unwinding, and breathing out totally.

In the event that you see any strain or snugness in your body, inhale into that piece of your body, and as you breathe out, experience yourself as progressively loose, quieter. On the off chance that contemplations enter your psyche, just notice them, and as you breathe out to let them go, proceeding to concentrate on your breath, taking in a more profound feeling of quiet and unwinding and breathing out totally.

Keep on concentrating on our breath as you enable yourself to completely loosen up your psyche and body, feeling a feeling of certainty and reestablishment filling your being. Experience yourself as loose, alert and sure, completely upheld by the seat underneath you.

Permitting harmony, satisfaction and certainty to full your being at this present minute as you currently open yourself to extending your experience of harmony and happiness. And now, as you experience yourself as completely present at this time, gradually and easily enable your eyes to open, feeling wide conscious, alert, better than anyone might have expected—completely present at this very moment.

Self-Love

Self-love is not just a condition of feeling better. It is a condition of gratefulness for oneself that develops from activities that help our physical, mental and profound development. Self-love is dynamic; it develops through activities that develop us.

When we act in manners that grow self-love in us, we start to acknowledge much better our shortcomings just as our strengths. Self-love is imperative to living great. It impacts who you pick for a mate, the picture you anticipate at work, and how you adapt to the issues throughout your life.

There are such a significant number of methods for rehearsing self-love; it might be by taking a short outing, gifting yourself, beginning a diary or anything that may come as "riches" for you .

Meditation for Self-Love

To start with, make yourself comfortable. Lie on your back with a support under your knees and a collapsed cover behind your head, or sit easily, maybe on reinforcement or a couple collapsed covers. For extra help, do not hesitate to sit against a divider or in a seat.

In the event that you are resting, feel the association between the back of your body and the tangle. On the off chance that you are situated, protract up through your spine, widen through your collarbones, and let your hands lay on your thighs.

When you are settled, close your eyes or mollify your look and tune into your breath. Notice your breath, without attempting to transform it. What's more, see additionally on the off chance that you feel tense or loose, without attempting to change that either.

Breathe in through your nose and afterward breathe out through your mouth. Keep on taking profound, full breaths in through your nose and out through your mouth. As you inhale, become mindful of the condition of your body and the nature of your brain. Where is your body holding pressure? Do you feel shut off or shut down inwardly? Where is your brain? Is your brain calm or loaded up with fretfulness, antagonism, and uncertainty?

Give your breath a chance to turn out to be progressively smooth and easy and start to take in and out through your nose. Feel the progression of air moving into your lungs and after that pull out into the world. With each breathes out, envision you are discharging any negative considerations that might wait in your brain.

Keep on concentrating on your breath. On each breath in, think, "I am commendable," and on each breathe out, "I am sufficient." Let each breath in attract self-esteem and each breathes out discharge what is never again serving you. Take a couple of minutes to inhale and discuss this mantra inside. Notice how you feel as you express these words to yourself.

On the off chance that your mind meanders anytime, realize that it is all right. It is the idea of the brain to meander. Essentially take your consideration back to the breath. Notice how your musings travel in complete disorder, regardless of whether positive or negative and just enable them to pass on by like mists gliding in the sky.

Presently imagine yourself remaining before a mirror and investigate your very own eyes. What do you see? Agony and pity? Love and delight? Lack of bias? Despite what shows up in the meditation, let yourself know: "I adore you," "You are lovely," and "You are deserving of bliss." Know that what you find in the mirror at this time might be not the same as what you see whenever you look.

Envision since you could inhale into your heart and imagine love spilling out of your hands and into your heart. Allow this to love warm and saturate you from your heart focus, filling the remainder of your body. Feel a feeling of solace and quiet going up through your chest into your neck and head, out into your shoulders, arms, and hands, and afterward down into your ribs, tummy, pelvis, legs, and feet. Enable a vibe of warmth to fill you from head to toe. Inhale here and realize that affection is constantly accessible for you when you need it.

When you are prepared, take a couple of all the more profound, careful breaths and, after that, delicately open your eyes. Sit for a couple of minutes to recognize the one of a kind encounter you had during this meditation.

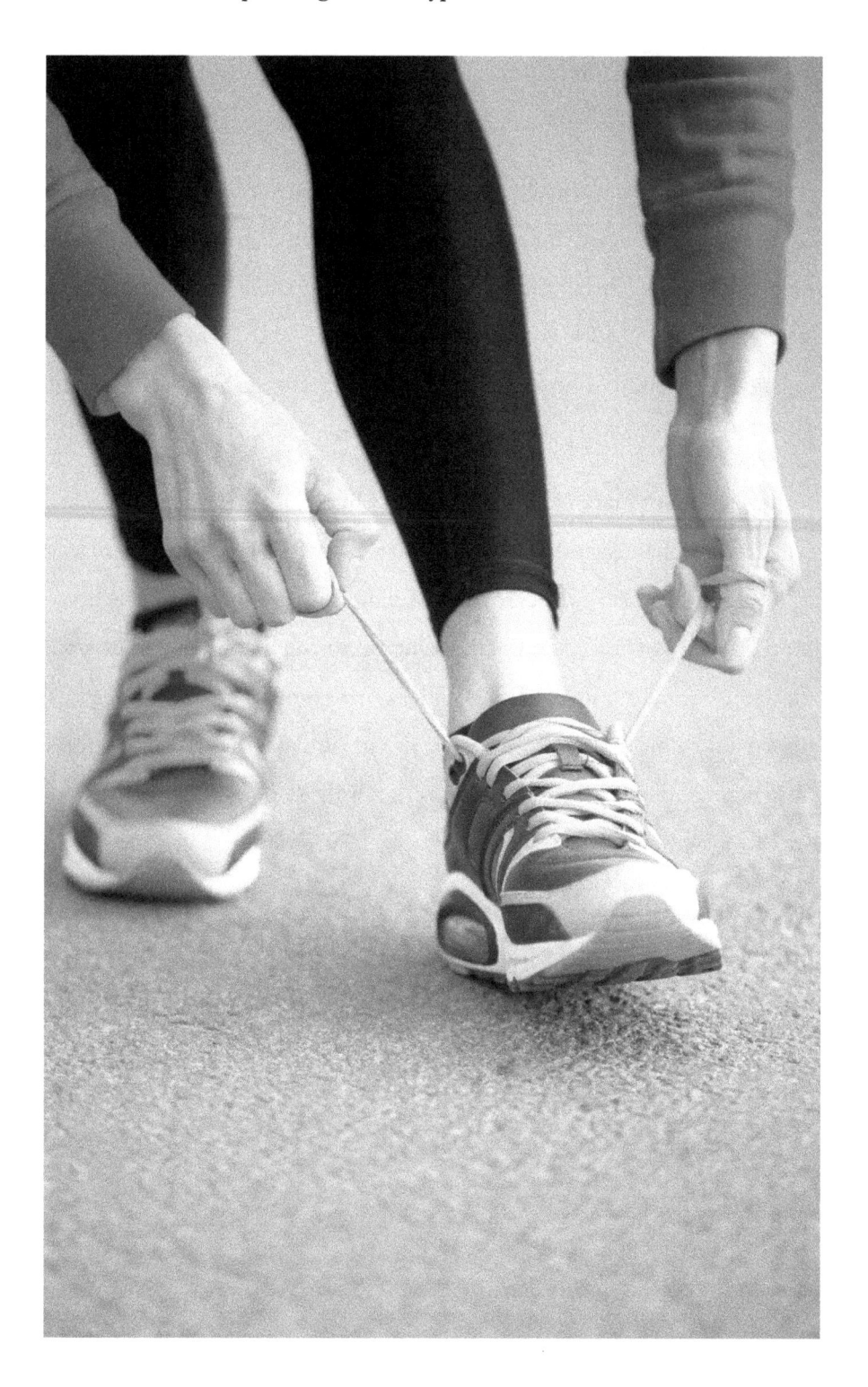

CHAPTER 5:
Pleasure Principle

Nutrition is closely connected to our sensory perceptions, and therefore to our memories. We remember how it looks, how we feel eating it, how it tastes. The tastes and textures of the food linger on the palate, from sweet to salty, crispy to crunchy, and take the mouth and mind to a happier spot.

It can be the smooth ice cream flavor that drives you—or the bittersweet chocolate abundance, the easy tart pop of fresh berries, or the crispy, chewy roast chicken goodness, or all of that, and more. Food tastes fine. This would be.

The enjoyment of taste, along with desire, is one of our essential eating motivations—a "spring," in terms of health-psychology. And still, flavor recognition is a double-edged knife.

Many people who struggle with weight and eating habits see their taste buds as their downfall. "If I could only miss the taste of the onion rings,

I think everything else will fall into place," said Lydia, 30, during one of our sessions, causing the rest of the room to laugh. "I am not crying!" It can sound counterintuitive, but learning to adapt to the taste of food will help prevent overeating and direct you to healthier choices. For example, distracted eating habits—eating really fast or watching TV, driving, or multitasking—short-circuit not only our hunger and fullness signals, as you discovered before but also our flavoring experience. So if you scarf down a Snickers bar from the grocery store on the way home, or eat a bowl of pasta and sauce in front of the TV, you barely notice what you're eating.

The subconscious always looks for gratification when this happens. What are you doing, then? Have some more. What's missing is a total eating experience, guided by the senses. The missing ingredient is not more food but focus.

We miss the feeling though, at the same time paying attention to other items. The answer, right? Remember to be mindful of every element of the food itself.

You will get flavor to work in your favor by learning to enhance your taste experiences. It offers you yet another tool in your toolkit for mindfulness.

Wired for Flavor

Satiety—the relaxed feeling that we have had enough food—causes us to avoid eating. We spoke about one sort of satiety, fullness. You have learned that one of the ways we know we've had enough food is through physical sensation—the way our bodies, particularly our stomachs, feel when we're eating or afterwards—and you've been practicing slowing down and tuning in to those sensations. One form of satiety is called "taste satiety," a phrase used by Jean Kristeller to promote comprehension of the idea of sensory-specific satiety. The satiety of the taste is not the mouth, but the tongue.

Eating food with a specific flavor—sweet, salty, sour, or bitter—builds peaks, and then starts to lose the enjoyment we get from it. The peak before decline is satiety of taste—the feeling we've had enough of a specific flavor. You know the sensation: the fourth cheesecake slice, when it goes from celestial to neutral.

Once the transition happens, the neuronal activity changes within the brain. Studies show that taste satiety in our hypothalamus, which regulates our appetite, and our prefrontal cortex, which regulates most aspects of our behavior, influences brain function.

A variety of factors affect taste satiety, including the size of the bites we consume, how physically hungry we are, how quickly we consume, whether we eat whole or processed food, and the flavor mix in each meal.

When it works normally, our mechanisms of taste satiety tell us that we have "had enough" of a specific flavor, but you need to slow down and pay attention to get the message.

Taste satiety is intended to promote interest in nutritional quality, eating a variety of foods. When you start eating hungry, you can usually hit taste satiety long before you experience fullness signals; when you eat a good, nutritious meal, taste satiety will help you consume some of the items on your plate. (It's more difficult to consume processed foods specifically engineered to overcome taste satiety, as we'll discuss below.) Knowing how satiety taste works is also a key to "pleasure eating"—those moments when you want something sweet after dinner or you're missing the salty, creamy taste of your favorite cheese.

The Physics of Flavor

Clients are always shocked by how easily when they slow down and pay attention to the flavor, they achieve taste satisfaction. With a single kiss, most achieve taste satiety, and after that, the flavor decreases. Understanding that from one piece of chocolate, you can get as much satisfaction as from ten is powerful knowledge, particularly when dealing with cravings.

Can you not stop taking a few bites with complete attention? For decades, scientists have been researching taste satiety, so there's a strong body of research on variables and techniques that influence how happy you are with a given meal or snack.

Although regular eating is rarely as attentive as in the above exercise, you can use taste satiety as a method for healthy eating by bearing in mind the following things: pace: the pace at which you eat will influence how happy you are going to be. In one test, which compared the experience of people consuming ice cream slowly (taking thirty minutes) versus quickly (in five minutes), consuming slowly led to significantly higher levels of a satiety hormone called peptide YY, or PYYY, for several hours after eating the ice cream. That suggests eating gradually keeps you happy longer—which can help reduce your total intake of food. Through our own clinical study and experience, we have found that you have to slow down the eating cycle and concentrate intensely to find differences in the taste.

Bite size: A cookie has the same calorie count, whether you eat it in three bites or ten. Yet how fulfilled you would feel from that cookie—and how much you end up eating—can differ dramatically, depending not just on your eating speed but also on the size of your bites. Which exactly is the explanation? Research shows that faster satiety is achieved, and less total food is consumed by taking smaller bites. Even if the caloric content is the same, more bites give you more sensory pleasure, so you get satiety of the taste faster.

Simple versus complex flavors: Studies and our clinical experience suggest that people with one flavor achieve satiety faster than with multiple flavors. Another groundbreaking research found that when people were given "pure sweet," like sugar water, on the third or fourth drink, they hit their taste satiety peak — much faster than you would expect. However, after many bites of a "pure" flavor like sweet or salty, some people do not tend to hit taste satiety, as described in "Taste Satiety and Weight Gain," below.

It takes longer to achieve taste satiety when complex flavors are involved, as they often are. Consider the salty-sweet blend of a Thai stir-fry, the combination of peanut butter and chocolate that has made Reese popular, or the dessert salted caramel phenomenon. When the flavors play in your mouth, your taste buds can start hitting sweet satiety but then get hit with salt, then back into sweetness, and so on. It's the difference between hearing a piece of music in its entirety (satisfying) and listening to three (confusing) overlapping tracks. The contrast is exquisite but often prevents the satiety of taste.

Whole vs. Processed: Research shows that foods that are highly processed take a long time to register in terms of taste satiety compared with whole foods. In other words, it takes a long time to feel relaxed even if you're eating slowly while you're eating flavored tortilla chips, frozen pizza with lots of toppings or a candy bar. It's not a disaster.

Food producers are well versed in taste satiety science and using it to their benefit, manipulating flavor and texture both to compensate for manufacturing processes that degrade flavor, such as dehydration and freezing, and to produce what is known as "hyper palatability." Manufactured foods—snacks, sweets, meals, condiments, and beverages—are sometimes designed to provide complex flavor combinations. And as you discovered earlier, you keep feeding when you're not full.

In other ways, too processed foods compromise our understanding of satiety. Food makers brought the sweet and salty tastes to a whole new stage, dosing processed foods with large quantities of artificial sweeteners and salt. If you regularly consume excessive amounts of sweet and salty food, that's what you expect if you consume, and your taste buds lose their sensitivity and need higher levels of flavor to reach the same satisfaction level.

There is proof that some of the sweeteners used in processed products, both calorie-laden types and low- or no-calorie sweeteners, do not register in our satiety center as natural sugars do, at a chemical stage. While glucose (natural sugar) is transferred through the brain and provides signs of satiety, high-fructose corn syrup, while caloric, does not reach brain tissue and thus does not signal satiety. In one recent research, the levels of PYYY and other satiety-related peptides did not alter when people were given the no-calorie artificial sweetener sucralose.

Processed foods are filled with sodium and artificial flavors, not only to produce a convincing taste, but also to disguise the bitter or bland aromas of chemical preservatives and other artificial ingredients. Participants do an exercise in our mindful-eating classes in which they suck the spice coating off a Dorito. They usually say there is no flavor in the chip underneath.

Processed foods do not need to ruin your taste experience forever, though. You can recalibrate your taste satiety back to a natural, balanced sweet and salty experience by moving to a full-food diet that provides more satiety per calorie than highly refined and processed foods. Because whole foods require more chewing than processed foods usually do, they appear to spend more time in your mouth. This increased "oral-sensory stimulation" may result in increased release of hormones in the gut satiety.

It will take time and patience to recalibrate your taste satiety, depending on how long you have eaten processed food and how much of it you consume. Working with hundreds of consumers over the years, we've found it takes at least two weeks to get comfortable consuming a diet that doesn't contain added sugar (and longer for a lower-fat diet). However, when you do, the natural sweetness of foods like fruit gets a lot more powerful.

Strong vs. Liquid: Approximately 18 percent of our calories come from beverages, many of which are high-calorie sodas, juices, sports drinks, and other canned drinks. Such "food calories" are a major culprit in the epidemic of obesity and a prime target for anyone who attempts to control weight. Nonetheless, a recent study by Johns Hopkins found that reducing calories from drinks contributes to greater weight loss compared with reducing calories from food. Here's what to bear in mind: while drinks can quench your thirst, they're not very successful at either satisfying hunger or satiety. If you eat liquids, natural processes of taste-satiety don't kick in the way they do with solid food.

CHAPTER 6:
Eating Out on Effective Weight Loss Program

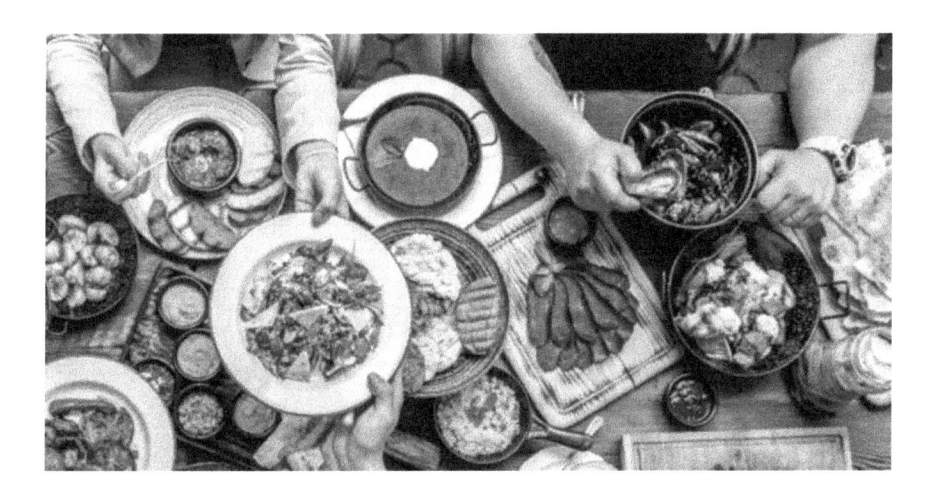

It is natural to worry about eating out, no matter what sort of diet plan you're on. There are moments when you're going to want to go out to eat to celebrate or hang out with friends, but you're concerned about finding entries that will fit inside your diet plan and still have all the tastes you want.

A successful weight loss plan is designed to help you eat based on your day-to-day daily activities. And that involves making the day that you go out to eat in order to enjoy life or do something a little special. So long as you are mindful of the food you eat when you go out, you can enjoy yourself when you go to your favorite restaurants. You're always going to have to be careful about your point values and be careful about going over or eating food that's too far from your limits and you're going to be all right .

Specific Rules for Eating Out

Every time you eat on a diet plan, you need to make sure you follow some basic guidelines that will make eating anything you enjoy easier, without having to go over your budget. Some of the guidelines you should follow to make sure you keep your diet promises:

Set a budget for food - you can set the budget for what you're supposed to do when you're going to the restaurant. How many points do you reserve for yourself, and how do you remain under this cap when you get there? When you want to know where you are going to eat in advance, you can look up some of the options before you even go.

Set the parameters early - set down the rules you are going to follow before you even go to the restaurant. Will you let yourself have an appetizer or a snack, or will you just stick to the main entrance? Was it possible to eat in the salad bar? Which sides do you allow yourself to be in? Using these instructions from the outset will help you stay on track and make this phase of decision-making simpler when you arrive at the restaurant.

Make special requests - most restaurants are used to special requests, so don't be afraid to ask questions. As long as you're not going too wild, most chefs would be able to make some changes for you.

For instance, you can ask that the sauce be put on the side of your meal instead of on the main entrance. Instead of frying it, you can ask to grill the meat or go with mixed greens as the side instead of the fries or another side, which isn't as healthy.

Go for portion control - if you're really looking at the portion sizes available in restaurants, you will find these can be at least twice as large as a regular meal. So if you do anything mega-size or add on, you make the portion sizes even more insane. There are a few things you can do to make sure you keep an eye on your parts.

One is taking half of the meal and putting it to go for later. This helps in preventing overeating when at dinner. You may select a salad, and then break the entrance into your group with someone else. You may also set up your own meal together, doing side dishes rather than the main meal together.

Learn the different terms - there are a lot of different terms that come up in the world of cooking, and each of them will mean different things for the points you use up when eating out. Grilled, steamed, and baked, for example, are usually healthier options, as long as there aren't many extra sauces added to the meal, while fried can be one of the worst.

Downsize - never get up while eating out from the smallest size. Each size you go up will add hundreds of calories to your diet, and several more.

Pick a smaller burger with several toppings, instead of a double or larger one with no toppings. If you can find a kids option instead of the big adult alternative, then go with it. Select smaller hands, or miss them entirely, if you can.

Look at the extras - the extras are always going to cut in your scores. When you add chips, cookies, something sweet or other things that aren't steamed vegetables, you'll consume more calories than you might imagine. Skip the bacon and cheese as well as the dressings as they add tons of calories, look out for double or larger sandwiches and even be vigilant of what things add to extra bread.

Be cautious with the toppings - salad bars are available in many restaurants, so filling up a bit on a salad and then having a smaller entrance to save points is a brilliant idea. Yet a lot of the salad bars come with a variety of toppings.

When you add a lot of these toppings, particularly with the dressings, to the salad, you cut into some of the points that you should eat instead. Be sure that the toppings on your salads, burgers and other items are held to a minimum and go with something like lemon juice to top it off rather than a sauce .

Watch the drinks - specialty beverages are extremely high in calories, sugars, and other unhealthy stuff for health. You don't want to squander all your points on the drinks you choose.

It's better to go with something that doesn't have alcohol in it at all and nothing that might be called a dessert as these would be the ones with the lowest calorie count. Water is a good option, and if you do want the taste of soda without all the bad stuff, you can get even sparkling water. Green tea, or sugar free tea, is also a great choice.

Stop thinking you've got to clean the plate - many of us slip into the pit of thinking we ought to finish the whole meal because we paid for it. Just think about how many calories you ordered in that big meal. Typically it's way more than we need and the extra calories, and a range of unnecessary nutrients on the body can do.

The easiest way to learn is to eat just as much as you like. Feed gradually because the brain knows it is a good place to start when it is full. Another idea is to bag half of the meal before it even hits you so you won't be tempted to eat more than you need to.

Eating out while you are on a diet can be a challenge. You want to go out and visit some of your favorite restaurants, but you are afraid you won't be able to stick with all the hard work you do. Yet, a successful weight loss plan recognizes that you want to go out and spend time with family and friends.

The Rules of Working Out

That said, when you get going on a new exercise regimen, there are a few things you can keep in mind. These will help you get started and make sure you get the right kind of workout to suit your needs.

Firstly, the type of exercise you select will make a huge difference. To target your whole body, you need to be able to pick out a wide range of workouts. Cardio is the first form, and you should spend three to four days a week getting some of this into your routine, as it increases your heart rate and makes sure your heart gets some of the treatment it needs. Plus, the weight loss is really great because you can burn a lot of calories in the process.

That doesn't mean certain forms of workouts aren't important. Weight lifting can also be done a couple of days a week because it also strengthens those muscles. Your metabolism will burn much faster during the day while doing normal activities when the muscles are toned up. So while you may not burn as many calories as you do with cardio during the actual workout part, weight lifting can be amazing for the metabolism benefits.

And on stretching you can't forget. Take some time off your days, and do some stretching, like yoga or some other technique. This can help give the muscles a good time to relax after having worked so hard during the week, make them stronger and leaner and prevent injury.

Now, when it comes to how long you're supposed to work out, that will vary. When you want to lose weight, it's recommended you work out at least three days a week for 45 to 60 minutes. However, some people prefer to work out at whatever minutes for five or six days, so it's easier to fit into their schedule. When you are just beginning your fitness routine and it's been a while since you've worked out, beginning slow is best. Ten minutes is better than nothing, and from there, you can build up. Never say you don't have time to work out; you can fit three or four ten-minute sessions into the day, and you've completed a full workout once you've done it.

Make sure the workouts you select have a lot of variety. Mix the stretching, cardio, and weight-lifting days together. Test out a host of different things, including some you've never done before. Mixing it up helps to focus on various muscle groups that helps with weight loss and can make your workout easier to enjoy.

Rapid Weight Loss Hypnosis Crash Course

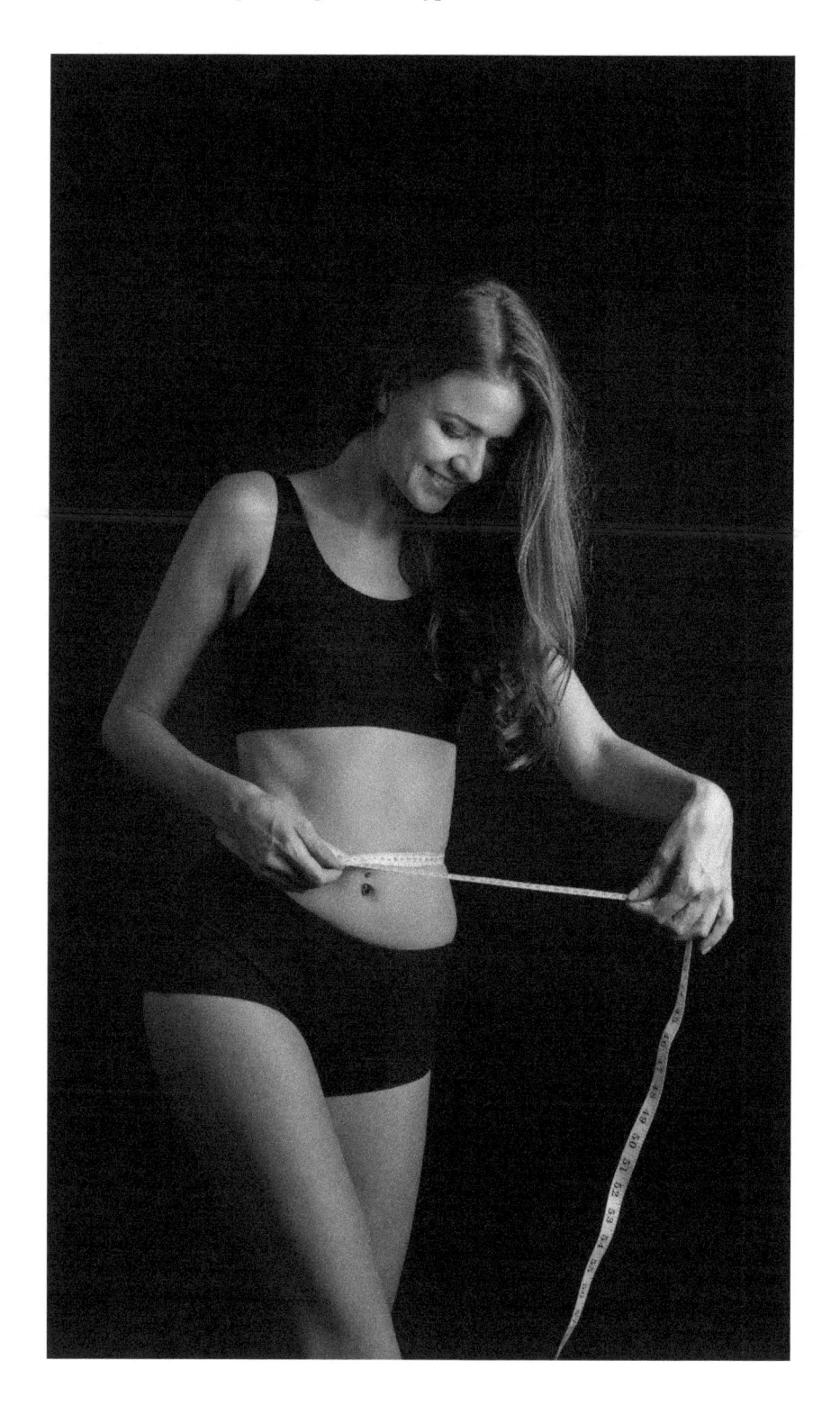

CHAPTER 7:

Foods to Eat for Deeper Meditation

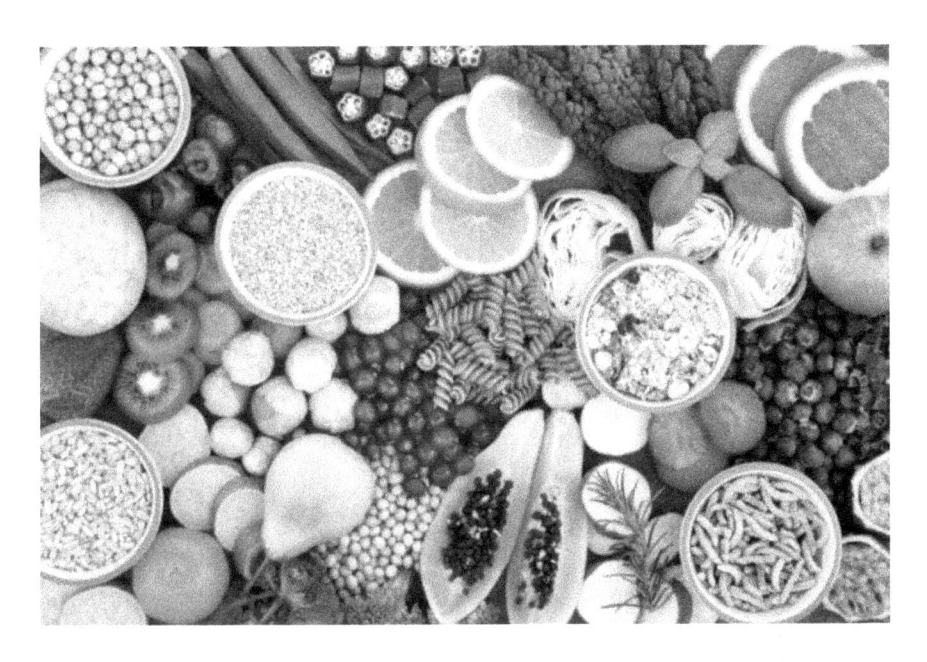

editation can be extreme. Take out every single stray idea? Concentrate just on your breath? Sit still for (at least) 10 minutes one after another?

In any case, we are finding out increasingly more that rehearsing everyday meditation has such a large number of astonishing advantages, from helping us become progressively empathetic to empowering us to be increasingly quiet, adoring, happy, excusing and liberal. Fortunately, there are a few nourishments that we can begin to consolidate into our eating regimens, which can enable us to pick up that laser center we are hoping to encounter when we plunk down to think.

Green Tea

Numerous old societies related tea with long life and well-being. Actually, starting in China, it has been utilized as medication for a great many years. Green Tea has not exclusively been filling our mugs for quite a while yet has played a job as a key fixing in numerous a sweet. It has been the subject in various restorative and logical investigations to decide if it is since quite a while ago, toted medical advantages really convey any legitimacy.

Furthermore, they do. Green tea lifts mental aptitude and standardizes glucose, so tasting on a cup before you plunk down to ruminate can be a valuable practice.

Tomatoes

Tomatoes have a lot of vitamin C, which is generally viewed as valuable in bringing down your pressure. As per an investigation led in Japan, members who ate tomatoes in excess of six times each week had an essentially lower danger of framing discouragement. Specialists are as yet attempting to make sense of whether lycopene, the synthetic segment that makes tomatoes dark red, legitimately influences the psychological prosperity. What's more, there are such a large number of approaches to appreciate them.

Nuts

Brimming with cell reinforcement Vitamin E and zinc, nuts, for example, almonds, pistachios, and pecans, are useful for boosting the insusceptible framework.

They likewise contain a lot of B-Vitamins, which help you oversee pressure and despondency. Scientists have demonstrated that nuts improve the capacity of our cerebrums to tackle issues, one more significant piece of meditation .

Vegetables and Whole Fruits

Eating an eating regimen wealthy in entire foods grown from the ground is probably the best thing you can accomplish for your body. The equivalent is similarly valid for the brain. Root vegetables, including sweet potatoes, squash, and carrots, are pressed with a wide range of nutrients and minerals.

However, the beta-carotene in these specific vegetables has been appeared to help your invulnerable framework to help keep you sound and keep your mind sharp. They are additionally crammed with fiber, which means they are delayed in their processing, and you will feel fuller more.

The most significant part of your meditation diet is that you start to consider nourishment to be vitality. Prior to eating, think about whether this nourishment contains the indispensable life power that you need. A few nourishments are loaded with vitality, and others will, in general, dull the psyche. As you ponder, you will become progressively delicate to what makes you feel better, and what cuts you down.

The more we can consider nourishment to be vitality, the more we will settle on savvy decisions in our eating routine. In any case, it is hard when we have spent our lives eating for eating. Attempt to see that all that you eat affects your body, psyche, and soul.

Affirmations to Heal Your Food Relationship

Our association with nourishment is personally associated with how sincerely protected, adored and sustained we feel. An expansion in craving may result from enthusiastic torment, the need to fill that excruciating, void spot with something.

The something you are truly searching for is love, yet in an apparent nonappearance of adoration, you manage with nourishment. An absence of craving can demonstrate a longing to withdraw from life, sustaining the hurt inside us again, showing a requirement for affection. Our association with nourishment can be perplexing. Incredible feelings of happiness and blame get into the blend.

By dispensing with your negative convictions about nourishment and your body that are never again serving you, you make space for a plenitude of positive affirmations that will serve you in tuning in to, trusting and respecting your body's individual needs.

Here is a rundown of affirmations you can include in your everyday schedule:

- I am the main individual who characterizes what well-being intends to me.

- I discharge myself from eating regimen mindset contemplations that are never again serving me.

- I respect the space between where I am now and where I need to be with my association with nutrition.

- I respect and trust my body and its needs by eating food sources that are pleasurable, fulfilling and supporting to me, and I give myself consent to appreciate all nourishments.

- I realize that I can confide in my body to give me the prompts and flag that will prompt adjusted smart dieting as a rule.

- Nourishment is not my adversary. I express gratitude toward it for supporting me and giving me vitality.

- My weight does not characterize my value.

- I value the extraordinary and remarkable qualities of my body.

- I discharge blame and negative sentiments I have about eating.

- I have everything inside of me that I have to feel totally free around nourishment.

- It is alright for me to tune in and trust my body.

- I pick self-care over restraint.

- I can be solid and cheerful at any size.

- I need to feel better and feeling great accompanies tuning in to my body and regarding its needs.

- I feel great consistently. Consistently, I advise myself that I can settle on the decision to feel better.

- Sustaining myself brings me delight, and I am deserving of the time spent on recuperating my association with nourishment and my body.

CHAPTER 8:
The Four Golden Rules

Even however you may have instant success with the hypnotic gastric band, it's significant that you use the Four Golden Rules that are the foundation of my system. They help to support the progressions you are making. You may ask why you need the golden rules since you have a hypnotic gastric band; however, in certainty, those rules are at the core of all the healthy eating of all naturally slim individuals. Naturally, healthy individuals eat when they are hungry, they eat what they need, they focus on their food and appreciate it, and they quit eating when they are full.

As it were, healthy, thin individuals follow the Four Golden Rules naturally. It is a natural, healthy approach to eat. The splendid thing about your hypnotic gastric band is that it makes the physical changes that make it natural for you to follow the Golden Rules as well. How about we remind ourselves of them now.

Golden Rule One - When You Are Hungry, Eat!

When a few people hear me state this, they believe it's crazy. They say, "That is the issue, I can't quit eating, now, he's proposing that I eat." What I am saying is that when you are really physically hungry, get yourself a healthy meal, and eat. If you starve yourself, your body goes into "survival mode," and you slow your digestion. So, when you are genuinely hungry, and you eat, your body knows there will consistently be sufficient food, so it doesn't slow the digestion, and you have enough fuel in your "body's engine" to do the things you have to do. It's critical to make the distinction between genuine physical hunger and emotional craving.

Real hunger starts gradually. It is clear and steady, and you feel it in your gut. It isn't activated by nervousness or by an emotional ache that goes ahead out of nowhere when you feel upset. It's anything but a response to fear, embarrassment, or outrage. It's anything but a plan to distract you when you are exhausted.

Real hunger is a straightforward physical feeling in your stomach. Sometimes, we confuse emotional distress for hunger. We suppose if we eat, we will feel much improved. Be that as it may, food doesn't fix emotions; it just covers them over incidentally. There are numerous, much better approaches to manage feelings than eating. If you speculate you need food because really you feel awful, you can use Havening to feel much better and afterward check in with your body and find whether you are actually physically hungry.

Recognizing Real Hunger

Proper physical appetite is a particular physical feeling, and with your hypnotic gastric band, you will think that it's simpler than at any other time to remember it. It will, likewise, be simpler to perceive when you are truly full. Be that as it may, for complete clearness and to ensure that you are precisely situated at both unconscious and conscious levels, I will request that you do a little psychological test that will help you in a split second and effectively perceive the signs for when you are really hungry and when you are full.

If you have ever endured your way through a diet, you will have contorted your reaction to your body's natural signals. This activity will push your mind to recalibrate your stomach's natural sensitivity to craving and satiety.

1.   Think about when you were super hungry—so hungry you felt swoon and even a crust of stale bread would have tasted delectable. Recall that.

2.   Now, think about when you were totally stuffed—when you'd ate and eaten so much food that you were in pains, even nauseous. Remember that.

3.   Do this a multiple time with the goal that you emphasize the contrast between being starving and stuffed

4.   Alright, now unwind. Those two feelings are the extremes. You never need to feel both of those terrible emotions again. You never must be that hungry, and you never need to feel that full.

I have created a scale where one signifies being so hungry you are about to blackout and ten signifies being so full you believe you will explode. It will assist you with recognizing effectively where your body is whenever.

The Hunger Scale

1. Physically blackout

2. Voracious

3. Genuinely hungry

4. Marginally hungry

5. Neutral

1. Six. Wonderfully satisfied

6. Full

7. Stuffed

8. Enlarged

9. Nauseous

Starting now and into the foreseeable future, NEVER go below three or over seven until kingdom thy come!

As you see, it gets simpler to live in the middle segment of the scale, your association with food, and your body will improve. You will feel more in charge, and like anything you practice for a couple of days, it will before long become natural. With your hypnotic gastric band, every one of these stages will be as clear as light. When you are somewhere in the range of 3 and 4, the time has come to eat. When you are somewhere in the range of Six and 7, the time has come to quit eating. With your hypnotic gastric band, you can't eat as much as in the past, so when you feel full, quit eating. Try not to attempt to eat more since it will sting to attempt to squash more food into your stomach.

Golden Rule Two - Eat What You Want, Not What You Think You Should

When you make food prohibited, it turns into everything you can think about. That is the reason for your gastric band, and with my system, there are no illegal foods. It's game over. You wind up having it and beating yourself. That method for eating resembles battling with your body. It resembles driving a vehicle by stalling the accelerator and pulling on the hand brake. It is a misuse of fuel, and it trashes the vehicle. This disorder is intensified by dieting. Dieting mutilates your body's natural systems. All diets include constraining and denying the body. So, the body's reaction is to hunger for high-energy crisis foods to make up the deficiency as fast as could be expected under the circumstances. That is the reason individuals on diets all fantasy about high-fat, high-sugar foods like cakes and chips and French fries and frozen yogurt.

The more they diet, the more they need those foods. There is nothing amiss with any of them, coincidentally—but as you move away from dieting towards balanced nutrition, you might be shocked to see that what you need to eat starts to change. As you become progressively touchy, food that you never focused on begins to speak to you. You will likewise see that you start to support new food, in any event, when it sets aside more effort to cook or get ready. This happens because your body is never again attempting to save you from starvation. It isn't searching for a crisis energy fix. Presently it is allowed to move towards more noteworthy well-being. As you lose weight, it searches out the protein, nutrients, and minerals it needs to fix and explain your skin and fabricate your muscles.

The extraordinary thing pretty much every one of these progressions is that you don't need to consider them by any stretch of the imagination. Your body's natural signaling system will control you. The more you focus on your body, the more you will understand that appetite isn't only a basic requirement for energy. You will start to see you are hungry for a particular food, for example, fish, or serving of mixed greens, or cake. You will see you lean toward one vegetable to another, etc. To summarize, dieters eat what a book discloses to them they ought to eat. Healthy individuals eat what their body truly needs.

Golden Rule Three - Whenever You Eat, Do It Consciously

This is potentially the most powerful suggestion I can give you, and what I am going to let you know is currently bolstered by various scientific research around the globe. When I state eat intentionally, I mean two things:

1. Focus on what you are eating, and that's it. Give your food your total attention. Concentrate on the food and NOTHING else!

2. Slow you're eating speed directly down. Slow down to about a fourth of your past speed and bite every mouthful multiple times. When individuals eat quickly, they flood their brains with happy chemicals (neurotransmitters), and they can't hear the signs from their stomach

that say, "You are full." So, they end up crazy and gorging. It's significant that as you bite every mouthful of food, you put your blade and fork down and bite your food 20—yes, 20—times!

If you can't do this, I don't think I can support you, and I don't want to believe anybody can. It's a little favor you can do for yourself that comes with an enormous reward.

Concentrate on Your Food

You can eat anything you desire, at whatever point you need, so long as you give it your total, full concentration. That never implies, at any point, eat, and do something different simultaneously. When you eat, sit at a table, eat your food from a plate, using a blade and fork, and chew your food multiple times. This may appear to be a little ridiculous to you now. However, it is completely indispensable to retrain yourself to focus on each mouthful you are eating absolutely.

This will guarantee that you truly make the most of your food. Appreciate the taste and texture of your food, and truly notice it as you swallow it and feel how it fills your stomach. By focusing on eating, you will think that it's basic and simple to notice the satiety signal that you get from your hypnotic gastric band, and you will quit eating and be fulfilled sometime before you would have expected to because you will feel how rapidly your stomach tops off.

This is the one thing I need you to do to ensure you can encounter the advantage of your hypnotic gastric band and get more fit. Conscious eating is the manner by which individuals forget about their body's natural weight control system in any case. By eating deliberately, you regard your food, and you regard yourself. Research has demonstrated indisputably that individuals consistently eat more when they sit in front of the TV. Concentrate on your food solely. That implies no TV, but also no perusing while you eat. Try not to surf the Internet or answer messages or reply to your friends. Try not to drink liquor when you eat, because it dulls your attention and diverts you from the real food. Try not to snatch snacks while driving or tuning in to music or playing a game or using your telephone.

That may sound demanding; however, it is likewise incredibly useful since it implies that you should just ever eat food that you totally appreciate.

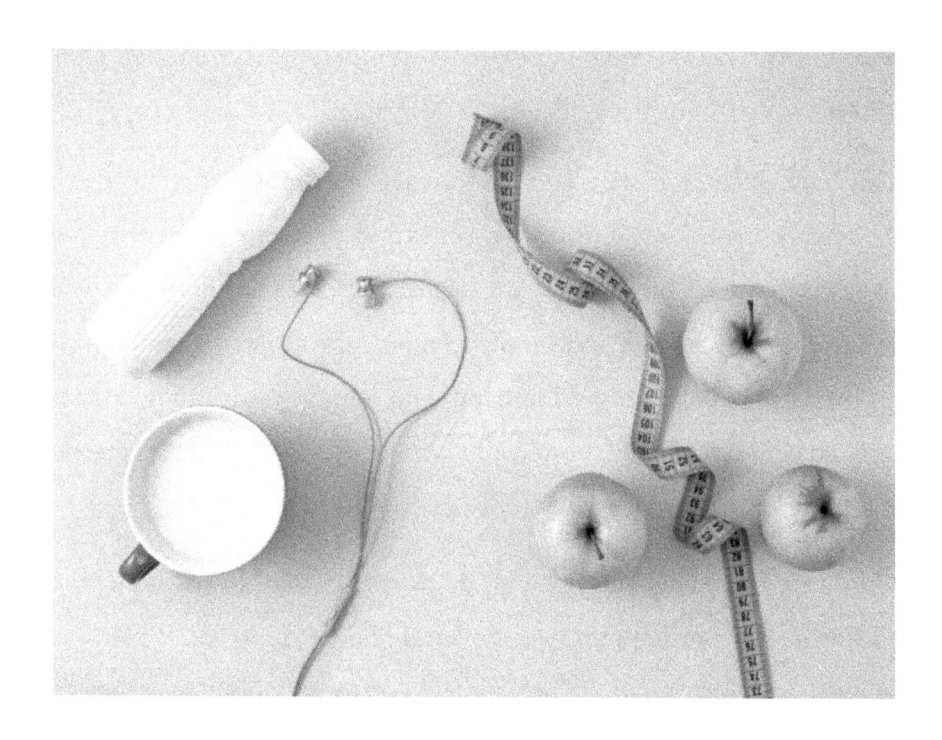

CHAPTER 9:
The Psychology about Weight Loss

Weight Loss Is Hard

As you already know, weight loss is hard. It's intimidating, and often doesn't feel good. You put yourself through hell at the gym, and you start to dread having to get up and go through the same awful things that you think are necessary for losing weight. Losing weight becomes a burden rather than a satisfying process, and with this mindset, even if you manage to lose weight, you won't feel good about yourself in the way that you should when it's all over because you'll be swaddled by negative feelings.

During weight loss, your body will often fight against you and urge you to eat more even though that is against your diet plan. Hormonally and emotionally, you'll want to go back to eating how you used to. Hypnosis can help stave off the urges, but it helps to understand what you're up against because this information highlights that dieting takes a lot more than willpower to be successful. You need to gather all your weight loss tools, and you need to use them to undermine the hardships of weight loss, or else you'll never find the success that you want and deserve. Weight loss isn't impossible, but it can seem pretty grim, especially in the beginning when you're still getting your footing.

The statistics are not on your side. Very few people actually lose weight. Just over forty percent of men and fifty-six percent of women in the world tried to lose weight as of 2019. A whopping sixty percent of high school girls have tried to lose weight. Many people are trying to lose weight in the world at any given time, but an estimated eighty to ninety-five percent of people regain weight after losing it. Often, this regain is attributed to unmaintainable weight loss regimes that are often advertised. Weight loss can be straightforward, but keeping your weight down in the long term can be arduous. The contestants of "The Biggest Loser" show this. While some contestants of the notorious weight-loss show have been able to maintain their weight, most returned to their original weight within six years.

People often focus only on the weight loss element of physical transformation, but thinking about just weight loss itself isn't going to lead to actual results. If people refuse to acknowledge the psychological impacts of weight loss, our weight loss statistics will never improve. There's so much misinformation out there about weight loss, information that tells people they need to starve themselves and subscribe to extreme diets. People are being set up by failure by diets that promise fast results but give no emotional support or strategies for maintenance. Eating well for a while isn't going to cut the cravings. You have to change your mindset if you want to change your life.

They aren't making genuine, lasting changes to their lives. Even so, to succeed at weight loss, you need to take measures that other people don't. Hypnosis is one such step, and understanding why you might be reluctant to give your all to lifestyle changes is another important step you need to take. So many people are afraid of changes, which is why fear is one of the biggest mental blockers that you have to defeat before you can lose weight.

Don't Let Fears Hold You Back

Fears can be so damaging to your progress. It's almost impossible to commit yourself in the way you need to if you are so fixated on your fears instead of what you can do to succeed.

Hypnosis is best done with willingness and openness, so don't let your fears hold you back and impede your ability to do what you've always wanted to do. Before you even start hypnosis, you need to analyze and understand what fears you have so that you can prepare for the major obstacles that will threaten your progress. Fears are valid; they stem from your brain wanting to protect you from danger, but you need to avoid overblowing them in your mind.

The fear of failure is one of the biggest fears that can disrupt your ability to give your all for losing weight. This fear can lead to you quit when you've only just gotten started. Nearly one-third of all adults in the United States have a fear of failure, and this fear can seep into every part of a person's life. It can make you feel insecure and unable to accomplish anything. This fear can make it hard to change anything too, and it can feel impossible to overcome the worry that you're just going to fail anyway. This fear can be draining because it makes you unhealthily obsessed with the things that could go wrong. Instead of thinking that you might succeed, you convince yourself that there's no chance that you will succeed. Then, you become a self-fulfilling prophecy and really do fail.

The fear of failure can easily lead to self-sabotage. When you fear failure, you'll avoid doing the things that could bring you success and choose the safety of stagnancy. You're not any happier by doing this, but psychologically, it feels safer. The truth is, though, that when you let your fears run your life, you're not better off because, in that scenario, you will never thrive. At least when taking a chance, you have the chance of triumph. When you have a fear of failure, you may subconsciously take measures to thwart your advancement. You will mess up, and then just quit because you feel like your progress has already been ruined.

You don't need to live with the fear of failure anymore. You can address this fear by knowing that you don't have to be perfect. You're human, and sometimes you're not going to do things in the best way. Hindsight allows you to see things that you didn't see before, and it can make you feel like a fool, but know that your mistakes don't mean you're a failure as a person. They are normal, and they are okay.

Look at your failures constructively. Don't even call them failures anymore because, more than anything, they are opportunities to grow. People often look at failure as something shameful, but when you have misfortune, it doesn't mean that you are incompetent or somehow bad. Use mistakes as a chance to grow. When you face failure, don't use that moment to give up or run away. Find ways you can improve. If you overeat one day, don't let yourself think that your whole diet is ruined because a good diet isn't shattered by one day of overindulgence. You need to understand that getting back on track is the biggest success you can have on this journey. For all the successes you have, you will have errors, but with a good outlook, those errors won't destroy you. They will build you up and help you learn through experience.

Imagine the worst that could happen if you put in a genuine effort. It's scary to think of the worst-case scenarios, but most of the time, the worst that you're thinking in your head is absurd and unlikely to happen. By letting yourself think of the worst that can happen, you can reduce the anxiety that you have regarding failure because the acknowledgment of what worries you is liberating.

By identifying what is truly bothering you, you take away the power of that fear and can prepare yourself for any disappointment or negative feelings that you may face on your weight loss journey.

Take the pressure off yourself. Putting yourself under pressure isn't going to help you. It's just going to stress you out. Try not to put strict time parameters on your weight loss. Don't tell yourself, "I need to be ten pounds lighter by the holidays," because the pressure is going to get in your head and make it harder to stick to your diet. It's okay to want to accomplish certain goals by certain times, but if those goals don't happen at the exact time you want them too, you must avoid being hard on yourself. Sometimes, things happen, and you can no longer meet the expectations you had for yourself. That's fine, and you can adjust your expectations accordingly.

Find aspirations outside of weight loss that makes you happy so that you have other things to keep you going when you have mishaps. Your whole life shouldn't be single-mindedly focused on weight loss. If it is, you're probably miserable. You have to have other goals to strive for that have nothing to do with your weight.

Find hobbies and activities that add excitement and happiness to your life because these will not only help you relax, but they will take your mind off food. It's hard to lose weight when you're thinking about food all the time, so let yourself think about other things. Be conscious about your dietary decisions, but don't allow weight to be the only thing that drives you.

The fear of not being enough, or the fear of being an imposter are also fearing that many people deal with. Many people think that no matter what they do, they will never be good enough for all the good things that they have. These self-esteem issues make it hard to find the incentive and momentum to lose weight.

The fear of not being enough often also feeds into imposter syndrome. Imposter syndrome is the fear people have in certain areas of their lives, especially work, that they are imposters who seem to be competent at what they are doing to other people but are just pretending to have the necessary skills.

They feel like imposters, faking their expertise to the people who they know, and they are terrified of being revealed as not worthy of what they have. People with imposter syndrome are perfectly competent, but they feel as though everyone else will see them someday as being ineffectual, which can result in these people avoiding attention and trying not to make any major changes.

To make yourself feel worthy, you can do a myriad of things, but the most important thing is to find enjoyment in who you are. See beyond what your body looks like or how well you do your job. Tell yourself that you are worth it. Affirmations are a smart way to convince yourself that something is true. Your brain believes all the things that you tell it most; thus, by repeating positive things about yourself, you will build worth and start to value yourself as a person more.

Be unafraid to be yourself. Don't keep the things you love and want a secret. Feel free to share what you love, even if other people won't necessarily relate to those things. Sharing your passions is an ideal way to bond with the people around you, and when you share your passions, you're reiterating that you are worth it by allowing the things you love to be validated.

Rapid Weight Loss Hypnosis Crash Course

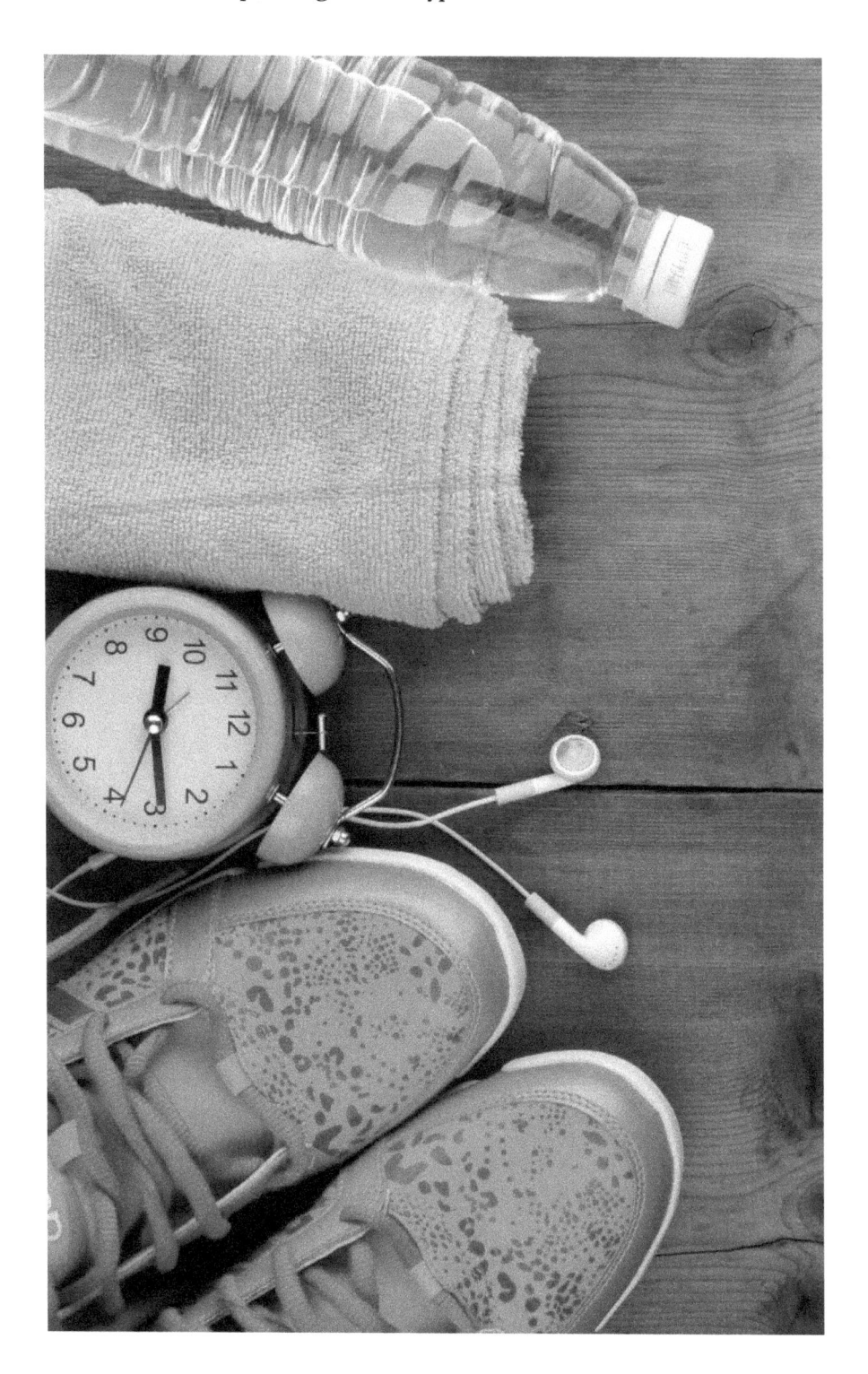

CHAPTER 10:

The Secret to Getting Rid of Weight Problems

What is the secret to getting rid of weight problems? I am going to tell you. The trick is breaking the old subconscious blocks, generating new patterns of thought and harmonizing the conscious and subconscious mind. Hypnosis will help you conquer the subconscious bloc obstacles.

You'll feel better. They're going to feel in control. You'll feel sure to be able to control your weight with encouragement and determination to keep up with your weight loss goals. Hypnosis has none of the negative or harmful side effects of diet pills or surgery. If you choose a successful diet and exercise plan and then reprogram your mind to make it no longer challenging but simple, pleasant, and efficient to follow your food and fitness programmer, you will certainly succeed.

Have fun exercising and eating healthy, so you can stop causing self-induced tension, stress, and discouragement. You will start doing the things that will help you in your aim of being safe and losing weight, obviously. You need to get rid of the unhealthy habits of thought that make you overweight. These thought patterns, which are stored in your subconscious mind, must be replaced with healthier thoughts and healthy behaviors so that you can instinctively do what you are expected to do without ever thinking twice about it .

Does that sound tricky? In reality, it's much less complicated than you would imagine. All you need is 10 to 20 minutes a day for a total of 21 days (the amount of time it takes to build a habit).

You can now have what it takes to speedily program your mind to lose weight. You see, hypnosis is one of today's world's most overlooked and powerful methods for self-change.

When you say "hypnosis," most people think of magic shows in Vegas or stupid acts on stage. Those on stage were chosen especially because of their susceptibility to suggestion. They wouldn't do anything that they normally wouldn't do on stage. For the publicity they receive, they really "do not mind" behaving stupidly on stage. If they don't perform, they know they're going to be taken off the stage and back to the seat. There could not be anything further from the facts. In theory, hypnosis is a very comfortable state of mind in which you become more receptive to suggestions. During the day, you usually go through hypnosis many times.

If the use of hypnosis for treating illness has been accepted by major medical societies, imagine how amazingly successful and beneficial it is when coping with thought patterns that stand in the way of the healthy body you deserve. The use of hypnosis has been used for more than half a century to treat illness. In addition, in 1955, the British Medical Association approved the hypnotherapy use. Its use was approved in 1958 by the American Medical Association.

In a 9-week trial-weight management group study (one using hypnosis and one not using it), the hypnosis group has continued to get results in the two-year follow-up, while the non-hypnosis group did not show any further results (Journal of Consulting & Clinical Psychology, 1985). The groups using hypnosis lost an average of 16 pounds in a sample of 60 participants, while the other group lost an average of just 0.5 pounds (Journal of Consulting & Clinical Psychology, 1986). Multiple studies showed that the addition of hypnosis increased the weight loss by an average of 97% during treatment and, more importantly, the efficacy increased by more than 146% after treatment. Hypnosis is known to perform much better over time (Journal of Consulting & Clinical Psychology, 1996). "The best way to break bad habits is by hypnosis," even Newsweek Magazine said.

Whether you want to use audio tapes or CD's for hypnosis, evaluate the script used to determine if the suggestions make sense to you. Make sure there are no negative suggestions.

The subconscious will not hear "no" or "don't," so the suggestion's emphasis would be: "I do not consume fattening foods." This will give you your objective in the opposite direction. Just use constructive feedback. "I just eat fresh foods that make me feel solid, safe, and happy" is much better.

How you perceive the suggestions is significant. If someone said, "That door should be closed," you get up and close the door or just think, maybe it should be closed and somebody else should close it. When you get up and close the door, it means you've "inferred" you're supposed to close your door. Some people don't like being asked what to do (direct suggestions). You may be making your own audio more effective. You might play a soothing audio, and then read or write your suggestions.

When you get up in the morning and before going to bed in the evening is the best time for your mind to accept these positive suggestions. You need a quiet room where nothing bothers you. When you're getting a lot of action in your house, you may need to find a room where you can shut the door and get undisturbed. It only lasts from 10 to 20 minutes.

Hypnosis is not a one-time fix for most people, the results are cumulative. The more post-hypnotic suggestions are applied to the hypnosis, the more permanent the results become. So, few people are likely to get hypnotized once to avoid smoking or lose weight. We usually create a new habit if they do, to replace the one they just quit. Most people who quit smoking begin overeating. We were replacing only one undesirable habit with another. Unless the root(s) of the problem is found, there would be no need to add another habit.

Having a specialist skilled in hypnosis and the weight-loss struggles could prove useful. Working with a specialist will help you understand the earlier programming and remove it.

Especially with weight loss, use the relaxation and self-hypnosis every morning and evening to be effective, changing and perfecting your suggestions while you lose weight. Upon reaching the weight you are comfortable with, you might want to add other goals along with strengthening your healthy eating and exercising habits.

You will need to start with full relaxation at first, but after a week or so, you will be able to go very quickly into the altered relaxed state by counting down from 10 to 1.

Always end your session with a suggestion that makes you feel good, better than ever, relaxed and either alert, clear-headed, refreshed, and full of morning energy or relaxed and able to soundly sleep when you go to bed at night.

Keep a pen and paper close by to write down any insights that come to mind while listening to your suggestions or reading them. You can recall things that you were told as a child that now influence your behavior. For me, I started to remember a lot of things I was told when I was a child that I never thought had bothered me until I was much older.

I just didn't connect those things that I remembered with my behavior. I became really mad when I recalled. I realized the life I missed by believing in what these people had said or taught me as a child and reinforced through the years by other people and events .

Weight Loss Affirmations: Are They Enough and How to Practice Them

Weight loss claims are one of the many daily affirmations people are practicing to improve themselves, but are they just enough to make a change, and how do you practice them effectively? This article discusses what to include with your positive weight-loss affirmations as well as ways to make them work.

First of all, when practicing affirmations of weight loss or any other affirmations of self-esteem, it's important to remember that you're "working from the inside out." What that means is that in order to make any change in your life, whether it's focused on your physical body or your finances, you want to change your mindset and inner mind (your subconscious) before any outer change appears.

While many people already know about this concept, it is not always practiced in such a way that positive claims for weight loss or other affirmations of self-esteem work as well as they might. You must really "believe" that you are thin in order to "be thin," and that is where most people "fall off the wagon" and avoid making their regular affirmations because the outer shift is not quick enough.

So, when you start, you decide to allow yourself enough time to make the inner change without any "expectation" of seeing any external changes.

Next, you will want to include other positive affirmations on a daily basis such as affirmations of self-love, spiritual affirmations, and assertions of faith and confidence. Why? For what? Because when you're trying to make progress, especially when it's about your own definition of yourself, you just want to "pour on love" to yourself and install as much "confidence" in the process as possible, and in yourself.

In fact, increasing your self-love and the ability to trust the process is critical for any self-affirmations to work on your list of affirmations because when you can increase your self-love, you have raised your "vibration" to the level of love that manifests things quicker. Often, you are more likely to view yourself better because you have greater self-confidence, and before you know it, you have lost weight effortlessly.

It is also important to trust the mechanism, because the vibration of confidence is absolutely necessary to attract what you want, which in this case is to be slim. And, by the way, it's vital that you don't use words like "don't" or "weight" when practicing weight loss affirmations, because they focus your mind on "what you "don't want."

"I don't want to overeat," for example, focuses on "overeating." On the other hand, affirmations of weight loss that contain terms like slim, attractive, fit, and safe are better options as they "rely" on being thin, attractive, fit, and healthy.

Creative Visualization

Once you find the right weight loss affirmations that make you feel great, get an image of the "perfect for your body" and place it somewhere around your bed so when you wake up in the morning you instantly see your target subsequent you. Then close your eyes and really "feel" when your body looks like that, and say your positive affirmations for weight loss and self-love affirmations.

The main thing to note at the beginning is that you want the inner change to happen first and affirmations are a great starting move, but self-hypnosis may be a better option to change your inner mind. However, self-hypnosis for weight loss is very common simply because it first works to change your inner mind which paves the way for outer change to follow .

Once you give yourself the time to make the inner change of seeing yourself thinner without any expectations of seeing the outer change actually becoming thinner, and you get the hang of visualizing your affirmations of weight loss that include affirmations of self-love and the ones of faith and trust, you'll be surprised how quickly you'll see the outer change happen.

CHAPTER 11:

Condition for Hypnosis to Work Out

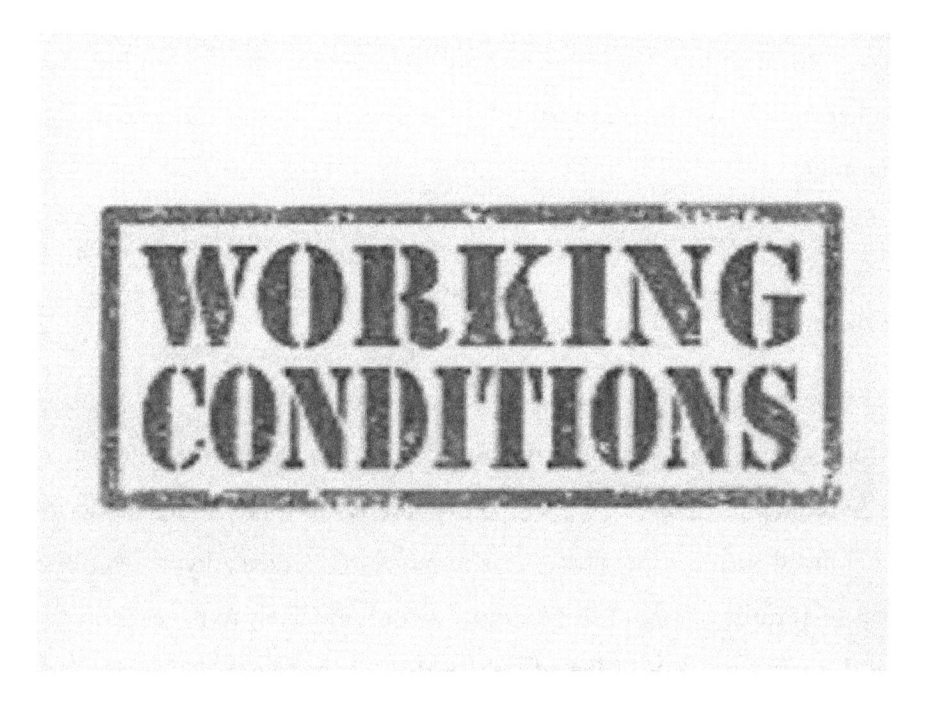

Although hypnosis itself cannot be accurately predicted, clinical experience and laboratory experiments at institutions such as Harvard and Stanford suggest that those who are most susceptible to hypnosis tend to share specific characteristics.

As already mentioned, virtually everyone can benefit from hypnosis. However, studies have shown that if you have most of these characteristics, you may be easier to hypnotize than others.

Here are some of the criteria for hypnosis:

Motivation

The motivation is at the top of the list. If you don't want to be hypnotized, you won't. If you are strong enough to change something, the chance is to be able to hypnotize yourself. But such motives must come from within. You need to want to improve yourself, not because other people think you should, but because it's what you need at the moment.

Optimism

Top people tend not to be skeptics if you take a continuum of hypnosis from low to high. This doesn't mean you can't hypnotize yourself if you're skeptical now. However, by the end of this topic, your skepticism will be alleviated somewhat so that you can experience hypnosis more easily. It turns out that most hypnotic people are likely to have a hopeful and optimistic view of life. To them, the bottle is not half empty but half full.

Defending

The people most susceptible to hypnosis are usually lawyers. This is an extension of buoyancy, trust, and hope reflected in their optimism. Whether it's something new in medicine, politics, art, or something that interests them, they are keen to spread the word. An opposite is a person who is very cognitive and very scientific in her evaluation. This individual demand evidence wants to read half a dozen books and scrutinizes the subject before committing himself. This attitude of the brain is not wrong. It merely means that such reality-oriented individuals must stay longer in hypnosis to get results.

Concentration

An important feature of hypnosis is increased concentration. Hypnosis deepens your concentration, but you need it to achieve this condition. The more distracting a person is, the more he responds to hypnotizing himself or is hypnotized by others. He also has to use this method more often to make a profit. Meanwhile, most people at least sometimes have a deep focus. Go to the room when they are reading and call their name. You can't get the answer. Those people can't hear your voice because they are too concentrated. We find no significant evidence difference between vigorous situation and self-hypnosis itself.

Acceptability

Many people are afraid to be hypnotized so as not to be absorbed in the will of others. This may be called Svengali syndrome. A mysterious stranger with a black cloak and flint's eyes seizes the soul of a naked girl while bending her will to adapt to an embarrassing wish. People who are prone to hypnosis have normal or good intelligence and a core of beliefs and firm attitudes that are fundamental to life. An example of such a person is someone with a well-trained religious education that embraces new ideas. He is hard to be fooled. He is sensitive to wise suggestions. Of course, the receptivity level differs from person to person. The receptivity for new ideas is one of the determinants of how easily you can get hypnosis. On a scale of 0-5 (0 is a person impervious to hypnosis), the majority of the population falls in the middle, for example, in the range 2 to 3. However, rest assured that your level of susceptibility to hypnosis is not included in the five-point scale. At the age of two or three, hypnosis should be repeated more often. However, being at the top of the scale has both disadvantages and benefits.

Imagination

Scientists at the Hypnosis Institute at Stanford University School of Psychology studied the hypnotic differences between individuals for nearly two decades. This is a project supported by the National Mental Health Institute and the Air Force Office of Scientific Laboratory. An organization that does not tend to fund trivial efforts. Dr. Josephine R. Hilgard, a clinical professor of psychiatry at Stanford University, reported that people who have been imaginatively active as a child could have hypnosis. The theory states that the imagination and ability to participate in adventures that emerged early in life remained alive and functional through continued use. Among university students, reading, drama, creativity, childhood imagination, religion, sensory, and thirst for adventure were activities identified as hypnosis. Hypnosis is deeply involved in one or more imaginary areas (reading novels, listening to music, experiencing the aesthetic of nature, adventuring the body and mind) can do.

Dr. Hilgard found that the student in major of humanities is most susceptible to hypnosis, the majors of social sciences are comparatively less, and students of natural sciences and engineering are not much hypnotized. The experience and research of other employees in this area tend to corroborate Stanford University results. According to Dr. Lewis R. Wolberg, a 40-year authority in the field: people with the ability to enjoy sensory stimulations and can adapt themselves to different roles have more tendency to be hypnotic than others.

Dr. Hilgard's lab was the most vulnerable to those who had fictitious friends in childhood and could read, adventure, and be immersed in nature. Suspicious, withdrawn, and hostile people have discovered that they tend to resist hypnosis. "Few people appreciate all of the above criteria. You don't even have to show improvement in all areas. You can make up for what's missing in another category. Defined these criteria, Hypnosis still needs a great deal of research, and the academic and medical community has accepted it as a subject worthy of serious investigation. A lot of eye-widening results are drawn from the study.

Rapid Weight Loss Hypnosis Crash Course

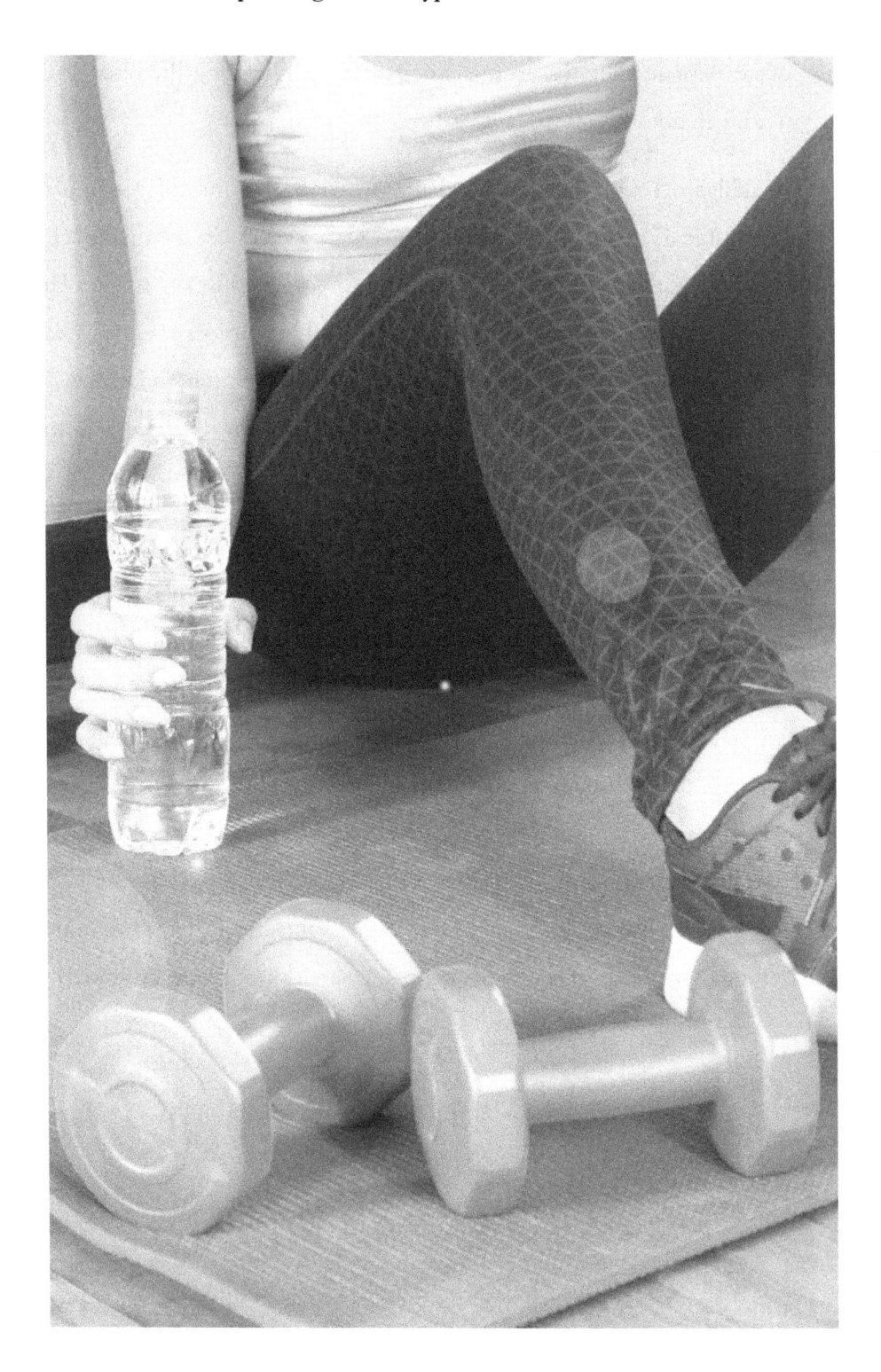

CHAPTER 12:
Your Thinner and Happier Life

Benefits of Eating Healthy and Detoxifying

Most times, we don't eat because we are hungry, we eat because food is available. The same way you make random decisions to purchase items you don't actually need in a supermarket in the same way that you purchase food. Most times, when you get a job that offers you some financial freedom, you begin to go to that expensive restaurant you have always dreamt of going because you can now afford it.

Now that you can afford the food there, you start to visit the restaurant frequently and purchase food that you do not really need. You are just buying the food because you have the money to do so, and the food is readily available.

Many of the bad decisions that make us eat food that we do not need to eat can be avoided if we start to focus our thoughts on getting what is necessary.

The process of getting that what is necessary requires you as an individual to be able to acquire some personal discipline. Before you purchase any food, you need to ask yourself if buying the food is really necessary. Ask yourself if the food that you are eating will add any value to your overall health. After asking yourself that question, you will know the right thing to do based on the response to the questions. It is an easy process to do, and it will help to save you from eating those carbs that only add unnecessary weight to your body .

Maintain a Healthy Body

Once we consume food, our bodies respond to what we have consumed. The response could be negative or positive. Different foods generate different feelings. You may not believe what some of these feelings are, except you focus your minds on realizing them. The power of meditation is that it allows you to be able to focus, concentrate on a certain thing that requires your attention.

This is an easy task to accomplish, and you only should evaluate how your body reacts to the foods that you are consuming. Once you eat some foods, you will notice that you feel energized, while some foods will make you feel tired.

Once you overeat, you will experience some sudden feelings of tiredness. You will begin to feel as if your body is too heavy, and so all you want to do is take a nap or a rest. Now when this happens, you should realize that it is a sign that whatever you ate was unnecessary, and hence the body will not use the food.

As a result, most of what you ate will become something that your body needs to eliminate. Thus, you will start to add extra weight, because the excess food in your body becomes excess fat in your body. On the other hand, if once you eat, it immediately makes you feel energized; it means your body was receptive to the food that you eat.

It means that your body was able to convert much of the food into energy, and each of those components present in the food will be well utilized by your body. This is beneficial for the well-being of your body, and it can help you when losing weight and prevent you from adding unnecessary weight.

Maintain the Bodyweight

Your eyes are shut. Envision coasting your desires ceaselessly. Envision what's pleasant for you to eat a day. Envision spellbinding helping you get in shape as the news seems to be. Psychotherapist Jean Fain from the Harvard Medical School gives ten trancelike recommendations to endeavor.

When I tell people how I make a lot of my life—as a psychotherapist who entrances thin individuals—they ask: Does that work? Typically, my reaction lights up their eyes with something among energy and unbelief.

A great many people don't comprehend that adding daze to your weight reduction endeavors can enable you to lose more weight and look after it. Spellbinding originates before the tallying of carb and calories by a few decades. However, this well-established technique for centering consideration presently can't seem to be completely held onto as an effective methodology for weight reduction.

As of not long ago, the real claims of prestigious trance inducers have been bolstered by insufficient logical proof, and an excess of pie-in-the-sky responsibilities from their issue kin, stage trance specialists, have not made a difference.

Indeed, even after a powerful reanalysis of 18 sleep-inducing studies in the mid-1990s demonstrated that psychotherapy clients who appropriately self-trance lost twice as much weight as compared to the individuals who didn't (and held it off in one research two years after the part of the bargain) unless if you or somebody you know has joyfully been constrained by entrancing to buy a crisp, littler closet, it might be hard to believe that this psyche over-body procedure can enable you to take a few to get back some composure on eating.

- **Seeing is thinking absolutely.** So, investigate yourself. To gain proficiency with a portion of the priceless exercises that trance must instruct about weight reduction, you don't need to be spellbound. There are ten smaller than expected ideas that are pursued contain a portion of the eating regimen modifying recommendations that my gathering and individual hypnotherapy weight the executive's clients get.

- **The power is inside.** Trance specialists believe that you have all you should to be effective. You truly needn't bother with an alternate accident diet or the ongoing suppressant of hunger. Thinning, as you do when you ride a bike, is tied in with confiding in your innate abilities. You may not recall how terrifying it was the point at which you previously endeavored to ride a bike. However, you kept on rehearsing until you had the option to ride, consequently, with no idea or exertion.

Getting more fit may appear past you moreover. However, it's just about finding your balance.

- **You see your conviction.** Individuals will, in general, do what they accept they can achieve. That is even valid for mesmerizing. Those fooled into deduction they could be entranced (for example, as the trance inducer proposed they would see red, he turned the switch on a disguised red bulb) demonstrated improved mesmerizing reaction. It is essential to hope to be made a difference. Give me a chance to propose you anticipate that your arrangement should work on weight reduction.

- **Highlight the positive.** Recommendations, for example, "Doughnuts will sicken you," negative or aversive, work for some time, however on the off chance that you need lasting change, you need to think emphatically. Specialists Herbert Spiegel and David Spiegel, a dad child hypnotherapy group, considered the most well-known valuable trancelike proposition. "I need my body to live in. I owe regard and security to my body." I elevate clients to create their very own energetic mantras. A 50-year-old mother who shed 50 pounds more rehashes day by day: "Superfluous nourishment is a weight on my body. I will shed what I needn't bother with."

- **It's going to come if you envision it.** Like competitors who are getting ready for the challenge, you are set up for a successful truth by picturing triumph. Envisioning a smart dieting day will enable you to envision the means expected to turn into a decent eater. Is it too difficult to even think about photographing? Locate a comfortable old photograph of yourself and recall what you did another way. Envision these schedules reviving. Or, on the other hand, picture acquiring direction from an older, more astute self later on in the wake of contacting her required weight.

- **Get rid of cravings.** Subliminal specialists utilize the intensity of emblematic symbolism on a standard premise, welcoming subjects to put sustenance desires on fleecy white mists or inflatables in sight-seeing and send them up, up, and away. On the off chance that you can direct off your eating routine from McDonald's brilliant curves, trance inducers comprehend that a counter-image can control you back. Welcome your psyche to flip through its picture Rolodex until you develop as an indication of yearnings throwing out. Push.

- **There are two preferred procedures over one**. A triumphant mix is entrancing and Cognitive Behavioral Treatment (CBT) with regards to getting more fit and holding it off, which patches up counterproductive thoughts and practices. Clients learning both lose twice as much weight without falling into the lose-a-few, recuperate-more trap of the health food nut. On the off chance that you've at any point kept up a sustenance journal, you've officially endeavored CBT. They monitor everything that experiences their lips for possibly 14 days before my clients learn mesmerizing. Each great trance inducer comprehends that raising cognizance is a principle move for the tyke towards suffering change.

- **Modify and then change.** The late pioneer of spellbinding, Milton Erickson, MD, focused on you. To change the lose-recuperation, the lose-recuperation example of one customer, Erickson recommended that she put on weight first before losing it—an intense sell today, except if you're Charlize Theron. Simpler to swallow: Modify your craving for high calories. Shouldn't something be said about some solidified yogurt rather than 16 ounces of dessert?

- **Like it or not, it is the fittest for survival.** No proposal is sufficiently able to supersede the nature of survival. Similarly, as we like to believe, it's the fittest survival, despite everything we're modified for survival in case of starvation. A valid example: a private dietary mentor needed a proposal for her dependence on a sticky bear. The advisor attempted to clarify that her body felt that her life relied upon the chewy desserts and wouldn't surrender them until she got enough calories from progressively nutritious food. No, she demanded, all that she required was a proposition when she dropped out.

- **Practice makes perfect.** There are no washboard abs delivered by one Pilates class, and one spellbinding session can't shape your eating routine. Be that as it may, discreetly rehashing a useful suggestion 15 to 20 minutes daily can change your eating, especially when combined with moderate, regular breaths, the foundation of any program of social change.

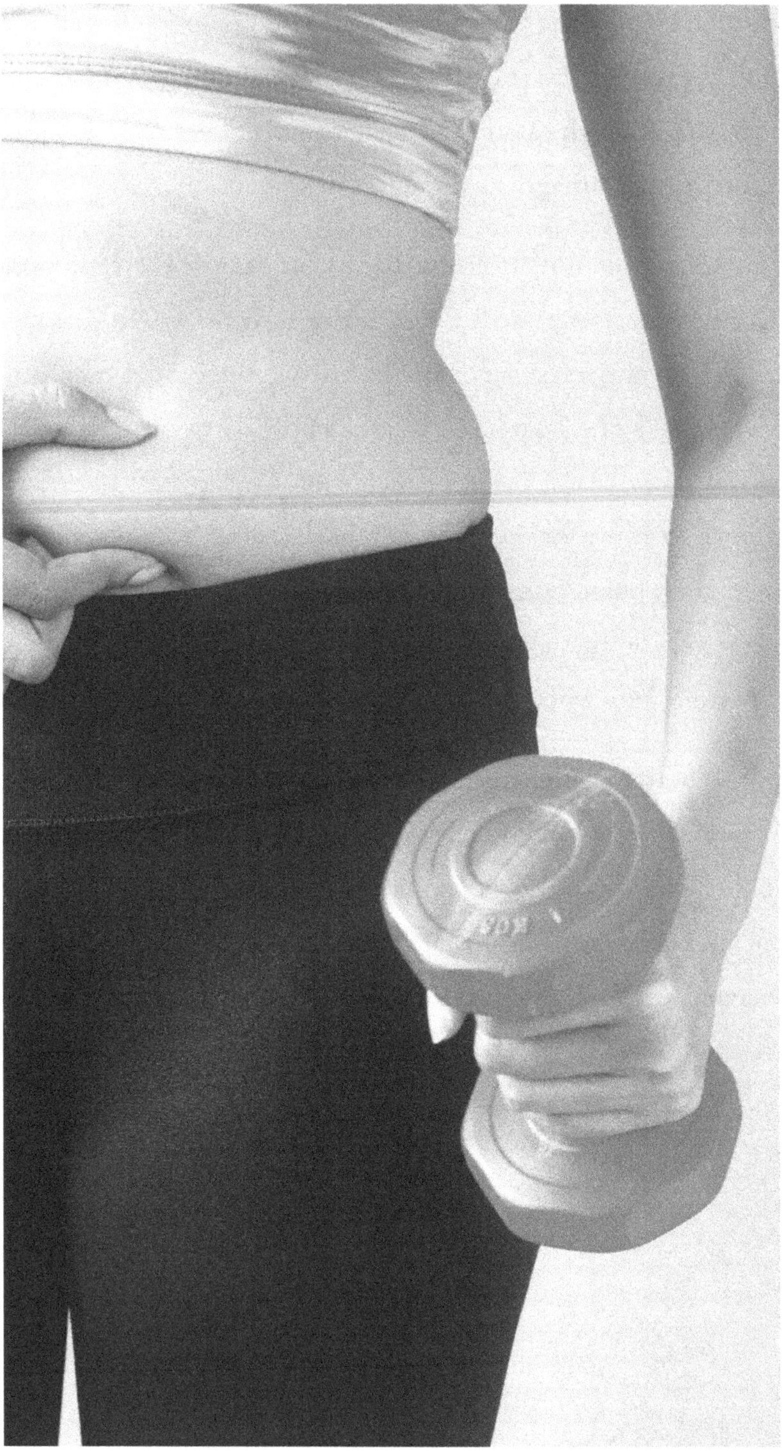

Conclusion

We went through how the nervous system is wired to hold onto trauma that is long forgotten by the conscious mind. But a tiny incident that reminds the body of that trauma can trigger a full-blown adrenaline and cortisol rush, set off a chain reaction or emotional eating and more stress just to make it impossible to lose weight.

We also shed some light on how abuse survivors subconsciously try to hide from the world by eating mindlessly and gaining weight. This is the protective function of weight that we discussed in the second chapter. So, it's evident how our subconscious actually never forgets the trauma of abandonment or abuse and turns I inward in a very dysfunctional manner.

Furthermore, a whole chapter was dedicated to introducing the concept of gastric band hypnotherapy. We started off by introducing the idea behind a hypnotic gastric band and its purpose, along with its key benefits and why it is better than an actual surgical gastric band. It is very important to know if the hypnotic gastric band will work for you or not, as it might not.

Thanks for reading!

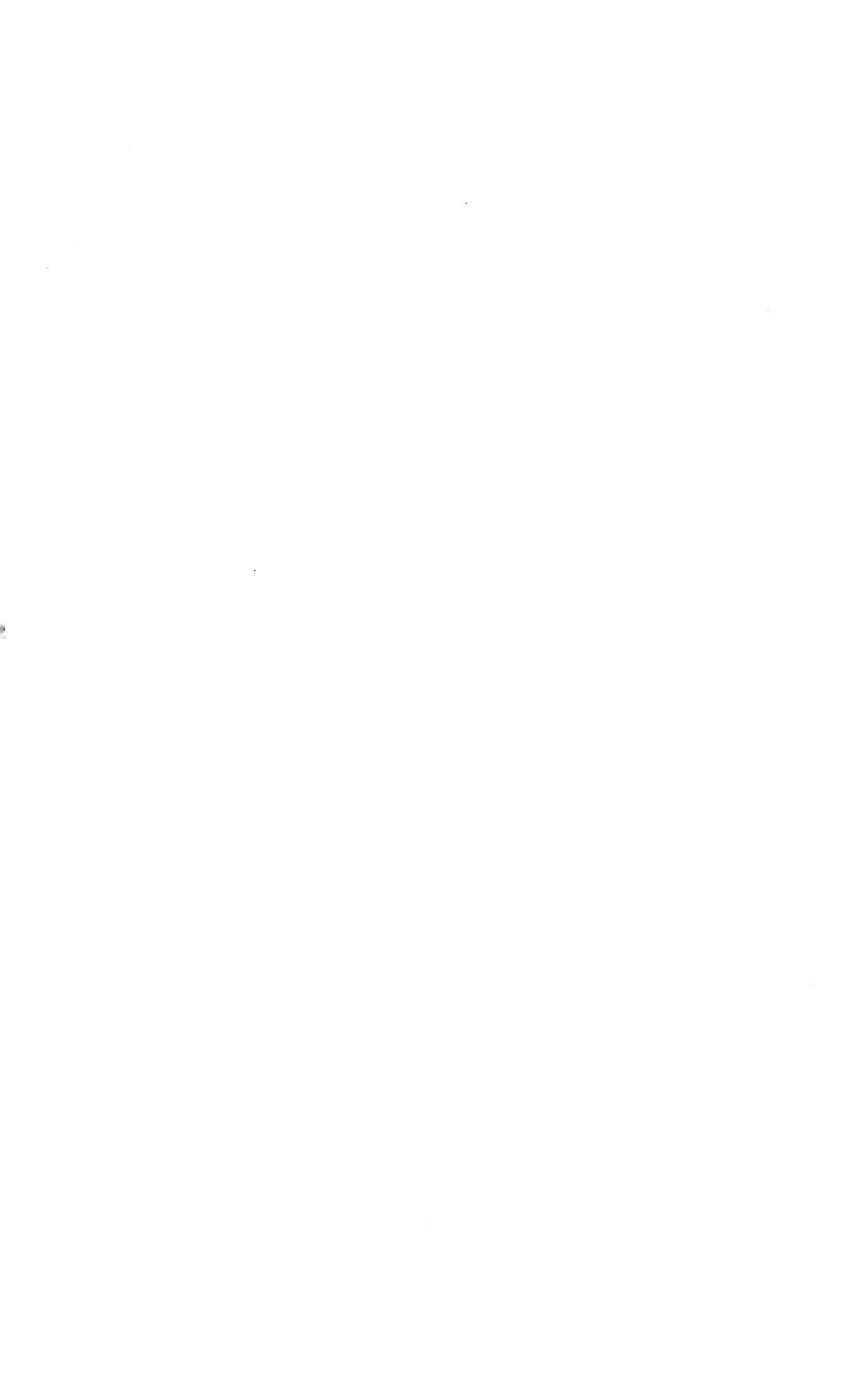